NATIONAL ACADEMIES *Sciences Engineering Medicine*

NATIONAL ACADEMIES PRESS
Washington, DC

Examining Glucagon-Like Peptide-1 Receptor (GLP-1R) Agonists for Central Nervous System Disorders

Convened September 10, 2024

Robert Pool, Eva Childers, and Sheena M. Posey Norris, *Rapporteurs*

Forum on Neuroscience and Nervous System Disorders

Board on Health Sciences Policy

Health and Medicine Division

Proceedings of a Workshop

NATIONAL ACADEMIES PRESS 500 Fifth Street, NW Washington, DC 20001

This activity was supported by contracts between the National Academy of Sciences and American Academy of Neurology; American Brain Coalition; American College of Neuropsychopharmacology; American Neurological Association; Alzheimer's Association; Boehringer Ingelheim; BrightFocus Foundation; California Institute for Regenerative Medicine; Cohen Veterans Bioscience; Dana Foundation; Department of Health and Human Services' Food and Drug Administration (R13FD005362); Department of Veterans Affairs (36C24E20C0009); and National Institutes of Health (75N98024F00001 [Under Master Base HHSN263201800029I]) through the National Center for Complementary and Integrative Health, National Eye Institute, National Institute of Environmental Health Sciences, National Institute of Mental Health, National Institute of Neurological Disorders and Stroke, National Institute on Aging, National Institute on Alcohol Abuse and Alcoholism, National Institute on Drug Abuse, and NIH BRAIN Initiative; Eisai Inc.; Eli Lilly and Company; Foundation for the National Institutes of Health; Gatsby Charitable Foundation; Harmony Biosciences, Huo Family Foundation; Janssen Research & Development, LLC; Lundbeck Research USA; National Multiple Sclerosis Society; National Science Foundation (DBI-1839674); One Mind; Paul G. Allen Frontiers Group; Simons Foundation Autism Research Initiative; The Michael J. Fox Foundation for Parkinson's Research. Any opinions, findings, conclusions, or recommendations expressed in this publication do not necessarily reflect the views of any organization or agency that provided support for the project.

International Standard Book Number-13: 978-0-309-73505-6
International Standard Book Number-10: 0-309-73505-X
Digital Object Identifier: https://doi.org/10.17226/29061

This publication is available from the National Academies Press, 500 Fifth Street, NW, Keck 360, Washington, DC 20001; (800) 624-6242; http://www.nap.edu.

Copyright 2025 by the National Academy of Sciences. National Academies of Sciences, Engineering, and Medicine and National Academies Press and the graphical logos for each are all trademarks of the National Academy of Sciences. All rights reserved.

Printed in the United States of America.

Suggested citation: National Academies of Sciences, Engineering, and Medicine. 2025. *Examining glucagon-like peptide-1 receptor (GLP-1R) agonists for central nervous system disorders: Proceedings of a workshop.* Washington, DC: National Academies Press. https://doi.org/10.17226/29061.

The **National Academy of Sciences** was established in 1863 by an Act of Congress, signed by President Lincoln, as a private, nongovernmental institution to advise the nation on issues related to science and technology. Members are elected by their peers for outstanding contributions to research. Dr. Marcia McNutt is president.

The **National Academy of Engineering** was established in 1964 under the charter of the National Academy of Sciences to bring the practices of engineering to advising the nation. Members are elected by their peers for extraordinary contributions to engineering. Dr. John L. Anderson is president.

The **National Academy of Medicine** (formerly the Institute of Medicine) was established in 1970 under the charter of the National Academy of Sciences to advise the nation on medical and health issues. Members are elected by their peers for distinguished contributions to medicine and health. Dr. Victor J. Dzau is president.

The three Academies work together as the **National Academies of Sciences, Engineering, and Medicine** to provide independent, objective analysis and advice to the nation and conduct other activities to solve complex problems and inform public policy decisions. The National Academies also encourage education and research, recognize outstanding contributions to knowledge, and increase public understanding in matters of science, engineering, and medicine.

Learn more about the National Academies of Sciences, Engineering, and Medicine at **www.nationalacademies.org**.

Consensus Study Reports published by the National Academies of Sciences, Engineering, and Medicine document the evidence-based consensus on the study's statement of task by an authoring committee of experts. Reports typically include findings, conclusions, and recommendations based on information gathered by the committee and the committee's deliberations. Each report has been subjected to a rigorous and independent peer-review process and it represents the position of the National Academies on the statement of task.

Proceedings published by the National Academies of Sciences, Engineering, and Medicine chronicle the presentations and discussions at a workshop, symposium, or other event convened by the National Academies. The statements and opinions contained in proceedings are those of the participants and are not endorsed by other participants, the planning committee, or the National Academies.

Rapid Expert Consultations published by the National Academies of Sciences, Engineering, and Medicine are authored by subject-matter experts on narrowly focused topics that can be supported by a body of evidence. The discussions contained in rapid expert consultations are considered those of the authors and do not contain policy recommendations. Rapid expert consultations are reviewed by the institution before release.

For information about other products and activities of the National Academies, please visit www.nationalacademies.org/about/whatwedo.

EXAMINING GLUCAGON-LIKE PEPTIDE-1 RECEPTOR (GLP-1R) AGONISTS FOR CENTRAL NERVOUS SYSTEM DISORDERS PLANNING COMMITTEE[1]

MATTHEW HAYES (*Co-chair*), University of Pennsylvania
BRIAN FISKE (*Co-chair*), Michael J. Fox Foundation for Parkinson's Research
LAWRENCE CHARNAS, Pfizer, Inc.
MATTHEW COGHLAN, Eli Lilly and Company
JON DAVIS, Novo Nordisk
EVA FELDMAN, University of Michigan
EDWIN (TED) GEORGE, Food and Drug Administration
SERENA JINGCHUAN GUO, University of Florida
ELISABET JERLHAG, University of Gothenburg
LORENZO LEGGIO, National Institute on Drug Abuse; National Institute on Alcohol Abuse and Alcoholism
IVÁN MONTOYA, National Institute on Drug Abuse
KIMBERLEI RICHARDSON, Howard University
LINDA RINAMAN, Florida State University

Health and Medicine Division Staff
SHEENA M. POSEY NORRIS, Director, Forum on Neuroscience and Nervous System Disorders
EVA CHILDERS, Program Officer
KIMBERLY OGUN, Senior Program Assistant
CHRISTIE BELL, Senior Finance Business Partner
CLARE STROUD, Senior Director, Board on Health Sciences Policy

Consultant
ROBERT POOL, Science Writer

---

[1] The planning committee's role was limited to planning the workshop, and the Proceedings of a Workshop was prepared by the workshop rapporteurs as a factual summary of what occurred at the workshop. Statements, recommendations, and opinions expressed are those of individual presenters and participants; have not been endorsed or verified by the Health and Medicine Division of the National Academies of Sciences, Engineering, and Medicine; and should not be construed as reflecting any group consensus.

FORUM ON NEUROSCIENCE AND NERVOUS SYSTEM DISORDERS[1]

DEANNA BARCH (*Co-chair starting September 2024*), Washington University in St. Louis
FRANCES JENSEN (*Co-chair*), University of Pennsylvania
JOHN KRYSTAL (*Co-chair until September 2024*), Yale University
SHELLI AVENEVOLI, National Institute of Mental Health (*starting September 2024*)
RITA BALICE-GORDON, Muna Therapeutics (*until December 2024*)
BRUCE BEBO, National Multiple Sclerosis Society (*starting September 2024*)
DIANE BOVENKAMP, BrightFocus Foundation
KATJA BROSE, The Chan Zuckerberg Initiative
TERESA BURACCHIO, Food and Drug Administration
SARAH CADDICK, The Gatsby Charitable Foundation
ROSA CANET-AVILÉS, California Institute for Regenerative Medicine
MARIA CARRILO, Alzheimer's Association (*until September 2024*)
MICHAEL CHIANG, National Eye Institute
TIMOTHY COETZEE, National Multiple Sclerosis Society (*until August 2024*)
BEVERLY DAVIDSON, University of Pennsylvania
M. DENISE DEARING, National Science Foundation (*starting September 2024*)
NITA FARAHANY, Duke University
EVA FELDMAN, University of Michigan
BRIAN FISKE, Michael J. Fox Foundation for Parkinson's Research
JOSHUA A. GORDON, National Institute of Mental Health (*until August 2024*)
DANIELLE GRAHAM, American College of Neuropsychopharmacology (*starting September 2024*)
MORTEN GRUNNET, Lundbeck
MAGALI HAAS, Cohen Veterans Bioscience
RICHARD J. HODES, National Institute on Aging
STUART W. HOFFMAN, Department of Veterans Affairs
YASMIN HURD, Icahn School of Medicine at Mount Sinai
STEVEN E. HYMAN, The Broad Institute of MIT and Harvard
MICHAEL IRIZARRY, Eisai Inc.
GEORGE KOOB, National Institute on Alcohol Abuse and Alcoholism

---

[1] The National Academies of Sciences, Engineering, and Medicine's forums and roundtables do not issue, review, or approve individual documents. The responsibility for the published Proceedings of a Workshop rests with the workshop rapporteurs and the institution.

WALTER KOROSHETZ, National Institute of Neurological Disorders and Stroke
ROBERT MALENKA, Stanford University
HUSSEINI MANJI, Oxford University; Yale University; UK Government Mental Health
HUGH MARSTON, Boehringer Ingelheim
BILL MARTIN, The Janssen Pharmaceutical Companies of Johnson & Johnson
DAVID McMULLEN, Food and Drug Administration
CAROLINE MONTOJO, Dana Foundation
JOHN NGAI, BRAIN Initiative
GENTRY PATRICK, University of California, San Diego
KATHRYN RICHMOND, Allen Institute
MARSIE ROSS, Harmony Biosciences
M. ELIZABETH ROSS, American Neurological Association
NATALIA S. ROST, American Academy of Neurology (*starting October 2024*)
KATIE SALE, American Brain Coalition
RAYMOND SANCHEZ, Bain Capital Life Sciences
TERRENCE SEJNOWSKI, Salk Institute for Biological Studies
JOAN SERENO, National Science Foundation (*starting September 2024*)
VIKAS MOHAN SHARMA, Neuraxpharm (*starting February 2025*)
SARA SHNIDER, One Mind
DAVID SHURTLEFF, National Center for Complementary and Integrative Health
JOHN SPIRO, Simons Foundation
ALESSIO TRAVAGLIA, Foundation for the National Institutes of Health
NORA VOLKOW, National Institute on Drug Abuse
CHRISTOPHER WEBER, Alzheimer's Association (*starting September 2024*)
RICHARD WOYCHIK, National Institute of Environmental Health Sciences
STEVIN ZORN, MindImmune Therapeutics, Inc.

Health and Medicine Division Staff
SHEENA M. POSEY NORRIS, Director, Forum on Neuroscience and Nervous System Disorders
EVA CHILDERS, Program Officer
KIMBERLY OGUN, Senior Program Assistant
CHRISTIE BELL, Senior Finance Business Partner
CLARE STROUD, Senior Director, Board on Health Sciences Policy

Reviewers

This Proceedings of a Workshop was reviewed in draft form by individuals chosen for their diverse perspectives and technical expertise. The purpose of this independent review is to provide candid and critical comments that will assist the National Academies of Sciences, Engineering, and Medicine in making each published proceedings as sound as possible and to ensure that it meets the institutional standards for quality, objectivity, evidence, and responsiveness to the charge. The review comments and draft manuscript remain confidential to protect the integrity of the process.

We thank the following individuals for their review of this proceedings:

MATTHEW COGHLAN, Eli Lilly and Company
UDI GHITZA, National Institute on Drug Abuse
VERONICA R. JOHNSON, Northwestern University Feinberg School of Medicine
SCOTT KANOSKI, University of Southern California
KAROLINA PATRYCJA SCIBICKA, The Pennsylvania State University

Although the reviewers listed above provided many constructive comments and suggestions, they were not asked to endorse the content of the proceedings nor did they see the final draft before its release. The review of this proceedings was overseen by **ELI Y. ADASHI**, Brown University. He was responsible for making certain that an independent examination of this proceedings was carried out in accordance with standards of the National Academies and that all review comments were carefully considered. Responsibility for the final content rests entirely with the rapporteurs and the National Academies.

Acknowledgments

The National Academies staff would like to express gratitude to the sponsors of the Forum on Neuroscience and Nervous Systems Disorders for supporting this workshop and other work of the National Academies; to the speakers whose presentations and remarks informed workshop discussions on the use of glucagon-like peptide-1 receptor agonists to treat central nervous system disorders; to the planning committee members for their time and effort in the development of the workshop scope and agenda; to Stephanie Eldridge (Spark Street Digital), Tunde Ogunfolaju (Spark Street Digital), and Caset Associates for their support in the broadcasting and transcription of the workshop; to Robert Pool and Billie Smith-Haffener for their writing and copyediting expertise and contributions, respectively, on this proceedings; and to the additional National Academies staff who provided critical support to the workshop and this proceedings: Christie Bell, Lori Brenig, Samantha Chao, Amber McLaughlin, Alexandra Molina, Marguerite Romatelli, and Taryn Young.

Contents

ACRONYMS AND ABBREVIATIONS   xix

1   **INTRODUCTION AND BACKGROUND**   1
History of GLP-1 Receptors and Current
   Therapeutic Applications, 2
Workshop Objectives, 4
Organization of the Proceedings, 4

2   **GLP-1 MECHANISMS IN THE BRAIN**   7
Highlights, 7
Overview of GLP-1R Circuitry in the Central Nervous System, 8
Mechanisms of CNS Penetrance for GLP-1R Agonists, 11
Discussion, 13

3   **LEARNING FROM THOSE WITH LIVED EXPERIENCES**   17
Highlights, 17
An Experience with Binge Eating Disorder and Obesity, 18
A Success Story of Using a GLP-1R Agonist To Lose Weight, 20
Discussion, 20

4   **INGESTIVE BEHAVIOR DISORDERS**   23
Highlights, 23
GLP-1R Agonists and Eating Disorders, 24
The Response of the Brain's Reward Regions to
   GLP-1R Agonists, 26

Binge Eating and the Endogenous GLP-1R System, 28
Discussion, 30

5 SUBSTANCE USE DISORDER AND ALCOHOL USE DISORDER   33
Highlights, 33
Preclinical Studies Examining the Effects of GLP-1R Agonists on Alcohol Consumption, 35
DPP-4 Inhibitors and Alcohol Consumption in Rats, 38
Preclinical Studies on the Use of GLP-1R Agonists to Decrease Cocaine Use, 40
Clinical Trials of GLP-1R Agonists for Treating Opioid Use Disorder, 42
Using Real-World Evidence to Study the Use of Semaglutide in Treating Substance Use Disorders, 45
Discussion, 47

6 NEURODEGENERATIVE DISORDERS AND OTHER EMERGING AREAS   51
Highlights, 51
GLP-1 Receptor Activity in Neurodegenerative Disorders, 52
GLP-1R Agonists in Treating Parkinson's Disease, 54
Penetration of the Blood–Brain Barrier by GLP-1R Class Drugs and Neuroprotectionm 56
Treating Idiopathic Intracranial Hypertension and Other Pressure-Related Disorders, 57
Biomarkers in Drug Development, 59
Discussion, 61

7 REAL-WORLD EVIDENCE, ACCESSIBILITY, AND HEALTH EQUITY   65
Highlights, 65
Using Real-World Data for Trial Emulation, 66
Shortages of GLP-1R Agonists, 68
Potential Barriers and Solutions to Widening Access to GLP-1R Agonists for the Treatment of Obesity, 70
Discussion, 71

| 8 | **WORKSHOP REFLECTIONS AND OPPORTUNITIES TO MOVE FORWARD** | 75 |

Highlights, 75
Panel Discussion, 77
Discussion, 81
Closing Remarks, 82

APPENDIXES
| A | References | 83 |
| B | Workshop Agenda | 93 |

Boxes and Figures

BOXES

1-1   Statement of Task, 5

7-1   Workshop Highlights, 76

FIGURES

2-1   The central glucagon-like peptide-1 (GLP-1) projection system, 9

3-1   Personal weight loss on Wegovy, 21

4-1   The CNS mesolimbic dopamine system, 27

5-1   GLP-1R agonist reduces alcohol intake in rodents, 36

6-1   Effect of exenatide on Parkinson's disease, 55
6-2   Effects of GLP-1R agonists on the central nervous system, 58

Acronyms and Abbreviations

AUD	alcohol use disorder
AUDIT-C	Alcohol Use Disorders Identification Test-Consumption
BMI	body mass index
CNS	central nervous system
CUD	cannabis use disorder
DPP-4	dipeptidyl peptidase-4
FDA	U.S. Food and Drug Administration
GIP	glucose-dependent insulinotropic polypeptide
GLP-1	glucagon-like peptide-1
GLP-1R	glucagon-like peptide-1 receptor
MOUD	medications for opioid use disorder
MPTP	1-methyl-4-phenyl-1,2,3,6-tetrahydropyridine
NIAAA	National Institute on Alcohol Abuse and Alcohol
NIDA	National Institute on Drug Abuse
NIH	National Institutes of Health
NST	nucleus of the solitary tract
PEG	polyethylene glycol

RCT	randomized controlled trial
TBI	traumatic brain injury
TUD	tobacco use disorder
VTA	ventral tegmental area

1

Introduction and Background

Glucagon-like peptide-1 receptor (GLP-1R) agonists have been receiving a tremendous amount of attention recently because of their ability to help individuals with obesity reduce their body weight substantially—up to 20 percent or more of total body weight in many cases (Campbell, 2023). First developed as a treatment for type 2 diabetes, GLP-1R agonists have been found to have promising effects in other disease areas besides obesity, such as ingestive disorders (e.g., binge eating disorder, bulimia, and anorexia nervosa), substance use disorders (e.g., alcohol, tobacco, opioids), and neurodegenerative diseases (e.g., Parkinson's disease, multiple sclerosis, and Alzheimer's disease) (Hölscher, 2022; Jerlhag, 2023; Jing et al., 2023; Kopp et al., 2022). In this rapidly evolving field, new and potentially effective applications are emerging frequently, making it challenging to stay up-to-date with the current state of knowledge.

To examine the promising yet understudied applications of GLP-1R agonists in neurological and psychiatric disorders, on September 10, 2024, the Forum on Neuroscience and Nervous System Disorders of the National Academies of Sciences, Engineering, and Medicine held a workshop, Examining Glucagon-Like Peptide-1 Receptor (GLP-1R) Agonists for Central Nervous System Disorders.[1] At the workshop, experts from a range of disciplines and perspectives reviewed the current knowledge and research gaps about the mechanisms of action of GLP-1R agonists and the evidence of their

---

[1] To learn more about the workshop, see: https://www.nationalacademies.org/our-work/examining-glucagon-like-peptide-1-receptor-glp-1r-agonists-for-central-nervous-system-disorders-a-workshop (accessed October 22, 2024).

1

clinical efficacy for eating disorders, neurodegenerative diseases, substance use disorders, and pain. Workshop participants also discussed the regulatory challenges and opportunities that may arise with the repurposing of GLP-1R agonists for central nervous system (CNS) disorders. This Proceedings of a Workshop summarizes the presentations and discussions from that meeting.[2]

HISTORY OF GLP-1 RECEPTORS AND CURRENT THERAPEUTIC APPLICATIONS

Glucagon-like peptide-1 (GLP-1) is an incretin hormone that has quickly emerged as being multifaceted and contributing to inhibition of food intake, proliferation of beta cells, and decreasing inflammation and apoptosis (Müller et al., 2019). Because of GLP-1's ability to decrease plasma glucose concentrations and revive insulin excretion, treatments that mimic this hormone, referred to as GLP-1R agonists, have been used primarily to treat type 2 diabetes and obesity (Collins and Costello, 2019; Hinnen, 2017).

Daniel Drucker, a professor of medicine in the Division of Endocrinology at the University of Toronto, began by sharing the history of GLP-1R agonists to treat various disorders. In the mid-1980s, he made one of the foundational discoveries, showing that GLP-1 directly stimulated insulin secretion and insulin gene expression but only when glucose was elevated (Drucker et al., 1987). At the same time, Drucker said, multiple studies showed the same effect in the rat pancreas, and soon after, clinical results showed that GLP-1 stimulated insulin secretion in humans. "We were very fortunate," Drucker said, "to have proof of concept translationally very quickly."

In 1996 three studies in rats and mice demonstrated that GLP-1 also inhibits food intake (Scrocchi et al., 1996; Tang-Christensen et al., 1996; Turton et al., 1996). Furthermore, if the GLP-1 receptor was blocked—with the GLP-1R receptor antagonist, exendin 9-39, or, in the case of the work in Drucker's lab, by using GLP-1R-knockout mice—the effect disappeared (Scrocchi et al., 1996). "So this was not an off-target, nonspecific effect," Drucker said. "This really was mediated through the GLP-1 receptor."

After those preclinical studies in 1996, it was not until 2014 that the Food and Drug Administration (FDA) approved the first GLP-1R agonist, liraglutide, for use in treating obesity in humans. Another GLP-1R agonist, exenatide, had been approved for type 2 diabetes in 2005. "So it took quite a while to go from bench to clinical approval," Drucker commented. But today, a decade after FDA approval of liraglutide to treat obesity, there are

---

[2] The planning committee's role was limited to planning the workshop, and the workshop summary has been prepared by the workshop rapporteurs as a factual summary of what occurred at the workshop. Statements, recommendations, and opinions expressed are those of individual presenters and participants and are not necessarily endorsed or verified by the National Academies, and they should not be construed as reflecting any group consensus.

many highly effective GLP-1R agonists available for clinical use, and dozens of these medicines are in clinical trials. "If you feel like you missed the last 30 years and you're getting into this late, we're really only just starting a new era of GLP-1 medicines in the clinic," Drucker said, adding that there are still opportunities for additional investigation.

Many different organs contain GLP-1 receptors, he said, which is why GLP-1R agonists are being explored for a wide variety of disorders, including metabolic liver disease, peripheral artery disease, cardiovascular diseases, kidney diseases, and disorders of the central nervous system (Drucker, 2024). The FDA's approval of liraglutide for the treatment of obesity has made it possible for researchers to collect useful data on cardiovascular and other outcomes in patients taking that GLP-1R agonist. And recently, clinical trials of such agonists have been carried out for a variety of conditions, such as heart failure with preserved ejection fraction, and renal impairment in people with kidney disease (Drucker and Holst, 2023). The result, Drucker said, is that a number of benefits of GLP-1R agonists have been well established for a number of different diseases or disorders. The most exciting to date have been the benefits for people with obesity, where tirzepatide has allowed many people to lose an unprecedented 20 percent or more of their body weight, he added, and understanding how all this works has tremendous potential for improving human health (Aronne et al., 2024; Garvey et al., 2016; Jastreboff et al., 2022; Wadden et al., 2023).

Another area where GLP-1R agonists have particular promise, Drucker said, is the central nervous system, which was the focus of the workshop. Some of the earliest work in that area came 20 years ago, when research using animal models showed that increasing expression of GLP-1 in the CNS was neuroprotective, while loss of function enhanced susceptibility to injury in the brain (During et al., 2003). Later, as large numbers of people took GLP-1 medicines for diabetes and then obesity, researchers observed that people taking these medicines had a certain amount of neuroprotection from other medical conditions such as stroke (Strain et al., 2022). Now, a number of ongoing and emerging clinical trials will test how well GLP-1R agonists can protect against Parkinson's disease, alcohol and substance use disorders, and other central nervous system disorders. For example, the agonists are being studied for their potential to control inflammation through the central nervous system (Wong et al., 2024), Drucker said, "and I think this is particularly relevant to understanding how GLP-1 might work in the brain." Other questions that Drucker mentioned need to be answered include: How many of these benefits in the brain and elsewhere are driven by reduction of inflammation? How many are driven by other mechanisms? How many are weight loss dependent? One recent cardiovascular outcome trial with the GLP-1R agonist semaglutide has indicated, for example, that at least some of the benefits may not be strictly dependent on weight loss (Lincoff et al., 2023; Ryan et al., 2024).

GLP-1 medicines do have some side effects, he said. Most of them are gastrointestinal, and, fortunately, these adverse effects tend to be reduced over time. On the other hand, the desired effects, such as enhancement of insulin secretion and reduction in appetite, do not disappear. Many of the effects are mediated through the central nervous system, Drucker continued, which is why the drugs are effective against maladies beyond diabetes and obesity (Drucker, 2022).

One exciting new front, Drucker said, is the new generation of GLP-1 medicines that activate multiple receptors, with tirzepatide being the first of what is expected to be a series of multiagonists. However, Drucker cautioned, every time something is added to GLP-1, it's important to consider whether GLP-1's effects are being preserved, enhanced, or offset. Those questions cannot be answered easily, he said, and answering them will require a great deal of work.

According to Drucker, "The future is unbelievably exciting. We're going to have different molecules and different delivery systems and different ways of manipulating GLP-1-based pathways, and the future is wide open for understanding how these might advance the therapeutic opportunity."

WORKSHOP OBJECTIVES

Matthew Hayes, Albert J. Stunkard Professor in Psychiatry and vice chair of basic and translational neuroscience at the University of Pennsylvania's Perelman School of Medicine, explained the workshop's four primary objectives (see Box 1-1). The first was to review the current state of knowledge regarding the mechanisms of action of GLP-1R agonists. The second was to discuss available scientific evidence on the clinical efficacy of GLP-1R agonists for treating various central nervous system disorders, specifically, eating disorders, neurodegenerative diseases, and alcohol and substance use disorders. The third was to examine the real-world evidence, accessibility, systemic challenges in health care access, and regulatory considerations surrounding the application of GLP-1R agonists as therapeutic treatments for central nervous system disorders. And, finally, Hayes asked presenters to highlight current research gaps and to consider opportunities to move the field forward.

Workshop co-chair Brian Fiske, the chief scientist at the Michael J. Fox Foundation for Parkinson's Research, reminded attendees that while they would be delving deeply into the biology of the field as they discussed the various aspects of diseases being targeted by GLP-1R agonists, they should keep in mind that there are real people who live with these conditions and deal with the effects in their daily lives.

ORGANIZATION OF THE PROCEEDINGS

Chapter 2 provides an overview of GLP-1R agonists, the GLP-1 system in the central nervous system, and the mechanisms through which the agonists interact with that system. Chapter 3 illustrates the human impact and significance of the work in this field with summaries highlighting the perspectives shared by individuals who have used GLP-1R medications. Chapters 4 through 6 examine the use of GLP-1R agonists in ingestive behavior disorders, substance use disorders, and neurodegenerative disorders and pain, respectively. Next, Chapter 7 tackles three topics pertaining to the widespread use of GLP-1R agonists: the use of real-world evidence such as electronic health records; the effects that rapidly increasing demand will have on the supply of GLP-1R agonists; and ways to encourage impartial and equal treatment of patients with GLP-1R agonists. Finally, Chapter 8 summarizes the key points and themes from the workshop as identified by workshop participants and potential opportunities moving forward. The references provided throughout the proceedings can be found in Appendix A, and the workshop agenda can be found in Appendix B.

BOX 1-1
Statement of Task

A planning committee of the National Academies of Sciences, Engineering, and Medicine will host a 1-day public workshop that brings together leaders and experts from academia, industry, government, philanthropic foundations, and disease-focused nonprofit organizations across disciplines (e.g., neuroscience, pharmacology, medicine, and endocrinology) to examine potential applications of glucagon-like peptide-1 receptor (GLP-1R) agonists in central nervous system disorders, such as dementia, Parkinson's disease, substance and alcohol use disorders, and pain.

Invited presentations and discussions may

- Review the current state of knowledge regarding the mechanisms of action of GLP-1R agonists and their therapeutic applications across different disease areas.
- Discuss available scientific evidence on the clinical efficacy of GLP-1R agonists, among other considerations, for treating various central nervous system disorders, including neurodegenerative diseases and alcohol and substance use disorders, and for pain management.
- Examine regulatory challenges and opportunities surrounding the application of GLP-1R agonists as therapeutic treatments for central nervous system disorders.
- Highlight current research gaps and consider opportunities to move the field forward.

A planning committee will develop the agenda for the workshop, select and invite speakers and discussants, and moderate the discussions. Following the workshop, proceedings of the presentations and discussions will be prepared by a designated rapporteur in accordance with institutional guidelines.

2

GLP-1 Mechanisms in the Brain

HIGHLIGHTS

- GLP-1 receptors are present throughout the brain and can contribute to a wide range of behaviors and conditions. (Drucker, Rinaman, Secher)
- Research is ongoing into which parts of the brain are directly and indirectly affected by GLP-1R agonists, but a complete understanding has yet to be achieved. (Rinaman)
- Experiments in rodents suggest that the endogenous central GLP-1 system contributes to metabolic state-dependent modulation of motivated behavior. (Rinaman)
- Although GLP-1R agonists can gain access to certain regions of the brain, this access seems to be through specialized uptake around the circumventricular organs, not through the blood–brain barrier. The precise mechanism by which this happens has not yet been explained. (Secher)

NOTE: This list is the rapporteurs' summary of points made by the individual speakers identified, and the statements have not been endorsed or verified by the National Academies of Sciences, Engineering, and Medicine. They are not intended to reflect a consensus among workshop participants.

OVERVIEW OF GLP-1 CIRCUITRY IN THE CENTRAL NERVOUS SYSTEM

Linda Rinaman, a distinguished research professor in the Department of Psychology and the R. Bruce Masterton Professor of Neuroscience at Florida State University, offered an overview of the central endogenous GLP-1 neuronal projection system. In addition, she described the distribution of the GLP-1 receptors (GLP-1R) and which ones may be accessible to systemic GLP-1R agonists.

To illustrate the central GLP-1 projection system, Rinaman showed a simplified version of the system in a rodent (Figure 2-1). The cell bodies of the GLP-1 neurons, which express glucagon, are located in the caudal hindbrain. They are split about 60–40 percent between the nucleus of the solitary tract and the intermediate reticular nucleus. The cells in the caudal nucleus of the solitary tract receive direct vagal sensory afferent input, and their axons branch widely to reach a large number of subcortical targets. Those targets include the midbrain, pons, hypothalamus, and limbic forebrain, including the amygdala and the bed nucleus of the stria terminalis.

If the GLP-1 neurons in the hindbrain are activated by physiological or pharmacological methods, or if the central GLP-1 receptors are activated, Rinaman said, this suppresses motivated behaviors such as food intake, drug self-administration, operant responding for drugs, and exploratory behaviors (Maniscalco and Rinaman, 2018). In rodent models, activation of the GLP-1 neurons also results in activation of stress responses, including anxiety-like behavior (Maniscalco and Rinaman, 2018).

Rinaman said that her laboratory discovered that the GLP-1 neurons in the rodent hindbrain are suppressed—that is, their ability to be activated is reduced—during states of negative energy balance, for example, after 18 hours of fasting in rats or mice (Maniscalco and Rinaman, 2018). The suppression of the GLP-1 neurons is accompanied by increased food intake, drug self-administration, operant responding, and exploratory behavior. "This is well recognized in people that [train] animals for operant responding for drugs," Rinaman said. "If you have them in a food-restricted state, they'll learn the task and perform the task much better." In sum, she said, "our working hypothesis is that the central endogenous GLP-1 system modulates motivated behavior, and it does so in a metabolic-state-dependent manner."

The axons of the hindbrain GLP-1 neurons innervate many subcortical brain regions, Rinaman said. GLP-1 neurons that target one region, such as the hypothalamus, thalamus, or bed nucleus of the stria terminalis, have axon collaterals that branch widely and reach every central target that is known to receive GLP-1 input, including the spinal cord. "So there doesn't

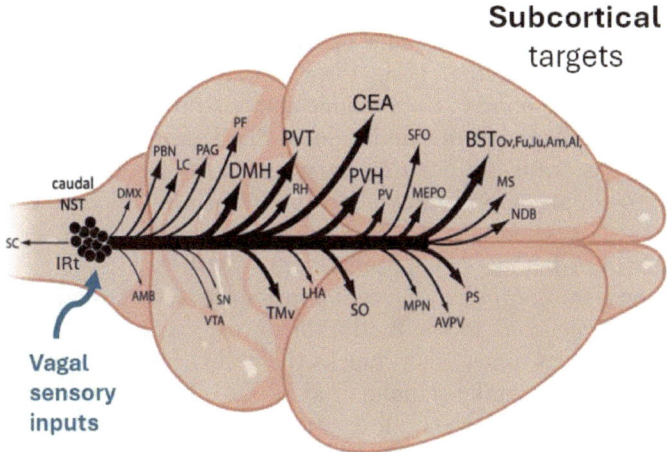

FIGURE 2-1 The central glucagon-like peptide-1 (GLP-1) projection system.
NOTES: The caudal hindbrain is located on the left. AMB = ambiguus nucleus; AVPV = anteroventral periventricular nucleus; BSTov,fu,ju,am,al =oval, fusiform, juxtacapsular nuclei and anteromedial, anterolateral areas of the bed nuclei of the stria terminalis; CEA = central nucleus of the amygdala; DMH = dorsomedial nucleus of the hypothalamus; DMX = dorsal motor nucleus of the vagus nerve; LC = locus ceruleus; LHA = lateral hypothalamic area; MEPO = median preoptic nucleus; MPN = medial preoptic nucleus; MS = medial septum; NDB = nucleus of the diagonal band; PAG = periaqueductal gray; PBN = parabrachial nucleus; PF = parafascicular nucleus; PS = parastrial nucleus; PV = periventricular nucleus; PVH = paraventricular nucleus of the hypothalamus; PVT = paraventricular nucleus of the thalamus; RH = rhomboid nucleus of the thalamus; SC = spinal cord; SFO = subfornical organ; SN = substantia nigra; SO = supraoptic nucleus; TMv = ventral part of the tuberomammillary nucleus; VTA = ventral tegmental area.
SOURCE: Presented by Linda Rinaman on September 10, 2024. Adapted from Gu et al. (2013).

seem to be a point-to-point, one-to-one subpopulation of cells that target different areas," she said.

The GLP-1 receptor is expressed in all these subcortical target regions and also in cortical and hippocampal regions that do not get axonal input from the GLP-1 neurons in the hindbrain (Randolph et al., 2024). Since the GLP-1 receptor is often present in the membrane of neural processes, including the axon terminals (Farkas et al., 2021), Rinaman said, it is possible that the GLP-1 receptor made by those cortical and hippocampal neurons is trafficked to their axon terminals in subcortical regions that do receive GLP-1 input.

Interestingly, she said, since the hindbrain GLP-1 neurons do not express GLP-1 receptors, they cannot be accessed directly by systemically administered GLP-1R agonists. They also, Rinaman added, get little or no synaptic input from neurons that express GLP-1 receptor in the nodose ganglion or area postrema. Thus, the vagal sensory neurons that express the receptor and respond to the systemic administration of GLP-1R agonists do not synaptically target the hindbrain GLP-1 neurons. Additionally, hindbrain GLP-1 neurons are not necessary for GLP-1R agonists applied systemically to suppress food intake. Nor are these GLP-1 neurons activated to express c-Fos when GLP-1R agonists are applied systemically (Brierley et al., 2021; Card et al., 2018; Secher et al., 2014).

However, she continued, a recent paper showed that ablating the GLP-1R-expressing neurons in the hindbrain dorsal vagal complex, including the nucleus of the solitary tract, blocks the ability of the systemic receptor agonist to suppress intake (Huang et al., 2024). Blocking the receptors in the arcuate nucleus or in the nodose ganglion does not block the effect, she said, "so we really need to focus on these hindbrain NST [nucleus of the solitary tract] neurons."

To address the issue of whether GLP-1R agonists applied systemically directly access central GLP-1 receptors, Rinaman showed some images of brain regions with GLP-1 receptors and the axons of GLP-1 neurons labeled in different colors (Farkas et al., 2021). The circumventricular organs, including the area postrema, are key areas where systemically administered GLP-1R agonists—and perhaps endogenous circulating GLP-1—have ready access to GLP-1 receptors, she said. There may also be access to some periventricular regions near the circumventricular organs.

A number of published studies have put a fluorescent tag onto GLP-1R agonists, including exendin, liraglutide, and semaglutide, and then used the fluorescent labeling to visualize the distribution of the agonist in the brain (see, e.g., Gabery et al., 2020). Rinaman said, "It could be that we're underestimating the amount to which these drugs penetrate just by virtue of the way those experiments are done and the non-enhanced visualization of the receptors." There are various reasons that the experiments using the fluorescent tags may underestimate the extent to which the GLP-1R agonists reach targets in the brain, she added. For instance, when a GLP-1R agonist is bound to a ligand, it promotes receptor internalization. Thus, there may be competition—if endogenous GLP-1 is already occupying a receptor, then the fluorescently tagged GLP-1R agonist may not attach and label it. Furthermore, since the GLP-1 receptors are trafficked and inserted into the axon terminal membranes, that may make it difficult to visualize binding, because one is looking at diffuse scattered axon terminals rather than concentrated neuronal cell body labeling.

Rinaman offered four key takeaways. First, the endogenous central GLP-1 system appears to contribute to metabolic state-dependent modulation of motivated behavior. Second, the hindbrain GLP-1 neurons are neither directly nor indirectly engaged by systemically administered GLP-1R agonists. Third, systemic GLP-1R agonists may access only a subset of the central GLP-1 receptors, including those in circumventricular organs and adjacent brain regions. However, current fluorescent imaging techniques may underestimate brain penetrance, and better techniques will be needed to get a fuller picture of which GLP-1 receptors are reached by systemically administered GLP-1R agonists. Fourth, GLP-1R protein is more prevalent in axon terminals than in neuronal cell bodies, and it is possible that endogenous GLP-1 and GLP-1R agonists may bind to GLP-1 receptors in regions beyond those in which GLP-1R mRNA is expressed.

Concerning research gaps and opportunities, Rinaman pointed to whether perinatal development of the GLP-1/GLP-1R system may help explain individual differences in responsiveness to GLP-1R agonists, why there are sex differences in the endogenous GLP-1/GLP-1R system and why GLP-1R agonists are more effective for weight loss in women than in men, and whether chronic exposure to GLP-1R agonists affects central GLP-1 receptors.

MECHANISMS OF CNS PENETRANCE FOR GLP-1R AGONISTS

Anna Secher, a scientific director within Obesity and MASH (metabolic dysfunction-associated steatohepatitis) at Novo Nordisk, discussed what is known about how GLP-1R agonists gain access into the brain. She began by reiterating something the previous two speakers had said—that interactions with GLP-1 receptors can play a role in various behaviors and conditions, such as appetite regulation and, potentially, neurodegenerative diseases, and that there are many different GLP-1 receptors scattered throughout the brain. Indeed, researchers have identified more than 50 brain regions with GLP-1 receptors, she said.

That raises the question of whether and how GLP-1R agonists, which were initially developed for use in the rest of the body, make their way into the brain. Molecules in the blood can get into the brain in three basic ways, Secher said. The first is by crossing the blood–brain barrier, which is composed of tightly connected epithelial cells. The barrier allows some small molecules to pass via diffusion and more active methods that transport desired molecules such as glucose or amino acids into the brain, but the barrier prevents most molecules and other substances from crossing into the brain. Second, cerebrospinal fluid has its own way of passing into the brain. Cerebrospinal fluid is produced by the choroid plexus and then secreted into the ventricular space of the brain; the choroid plexus contains a blood–cerebrospinal fluid barrier to protect the brain from potentially damaging substances in the blood. The third type of access is via the circumventricular organs, which include but are not limited to the median eminence in the hypothalamus and the area postrema in the hindbrain, and the pituitary gland. These organs have fenestrated capillaries, that is, capillaries with small pores that allow proteins and other large molecules to leave the bloodstream and enter adjacent organs.

To explore how well GLP-1R agonists access various parts of the brain, Secher's team labeled various agonists with fluorescent tags so that when they administered the agonists to mice, they could see which areas of their brains lit up. They found that although many regions of the brain have GLP-1 receptors, when the mice were dosed with the GLP-1R agonist semaglutide, the semaglutide ended up on only a fraction of the mouse brain's GLP-1 receptors, mainly in the hypothalamus, brainstem, and septum.

"So," Secher asked, "does that mean that these are the only regions that are activated by GLP-1 receptor agonists?" She and her team do not believe that this is the case, she said, "because when you have interaction with one neuron, this can communicate to many other neurons in deeper layers of the brain." To test whether that was happening, her team used c-Fos, a protein that can be used as a marker for neuronal activation. When they administered semaglutide to lab animals, the c-Fos distribution indicated that a number of brain regions were being indirectly activated by the GLP-1R agonist that had not shown up as being directly activated (Gabery et al., 2020). And, Secher added, since c-Fos is not a global marker, it is possible that many other brain regions were also indirectly activated by semaglutide but did not show up with the c-Fos signal.

Secher suggested that there may be limitations to the evaluation of the distribution and access of the GLP-1R agonists by the labeling method. GLP-1R agonists are internalized upon binding and are transported away from the region where they are binding. With this background, Secher addressed the issue of how GLP-1R agonists—and also antagonists—gain access into the brain. "We actually don't know yet," she said, "but we do have hypotheses." One of the hypotheses is that GLP-1R agonists gain access through interactions around the circumventricular organs. In addition to their fenestrated capillaries, the circumventricular organs also contain specialized cell structures called tanycytes, which send projections into the surrounding blood vessels and also into the brain parenchyma, that is, the brain's functional tissue, which comprises neurons, glial cells, and collagen proteins. These tanycytes have been shown to play a role in the access that leptin, a hormone that regulates the balance of food intake and energy expenditure, has into the brain through an interaction with leptin receptors. "We wondered whether that was the same mechanism with our GLP-1 receptor agonist," she said. To investigate this, they carried out an electron microscopy analysis with Csaba Fekete of the Institute of Experimental Medicine at the Hungarian Academy of Sciences and found that the tanycytes did have GLP-1 receptors. Other cells related to the blood–brain barrier did not have these receptors, Secher said. "This indicates that it's not a general access across the blood–brain barrier we have here with our

GLP-1 receptor agonist but rather a specialized uptake, likely around circumventricular organs."

She concluded with the following key takeaways: Both GLP-1 and acylated GLP-1 analogs have access to discrete brain regions. The access seems to be not through the blood–brain barrier but rather through a specialized uptake around the circumventricular organs. And the mechanism of how these molecules are taken up remains to be fully explained.

DISCUSSION

Cheryl Lohman, an independent researcher, asked whether GLP-1R agonists may be effective against long COVID given that inflammation is known to play a role in that condition. Daniel Drucker answered that it is a good question, but he knows of no rigorous scientific data that address the issue.

Endogenous Inducers of GLP-1 Release

Frances Jensen, a professor of neurology and the chair of neurology at the Perelman School of Medicine, University of Pennsylvania, and codirector of Penn Translational Neuroscience Center, noted that the focus in the field so far has been on administering GLP-1R agonists, but there are other ways that one could trigger the release of GLP-1. "What are other endogenous inducers of endogenous GLP-1 release," she asked, "and why has that not been a pathway for pharmaceutical development?"

Drucker answered that this is still an area of investigation, but it has received less attention given the effectiveness of GLP-1R agonists. "I think the bump in the road was really the development of oral semaglutide, which showed that you could give oral GLP-1 and have pretty impressive pharmaceutical activity," he said. "Novo Nordisk has demonstrated that you can get 50 milligrams of oral semaglutide in new formulation and have 15 percent body weight loss." It is not easy to achieve the same level of GLP-1 secretion with other approaches, he said, but some companies are still working to develop effective GLP-1 secretagogues, or substances that cause GLP-1 to be secreted, he said. "It's just much harder for them to be competitive in the new era of small-molecule GLP-1 receptor agonists, oral peptide therapeutics." Secher added that there may be a physiological limit to the amount of GLP-1 that can be produced with endogenous inducers of endogenous GLP-1 release compared with pharmacological inducers.

Brian Fiske asked Rinaman about the role of brain-derived GLP-1. Rinaman explained that when GLP-1R agonist drugs are given systemically, they are not recruiting the central GLP-1 endogenous neurons but are accessing a subset of the receptors. "Under the circumstances where the GLP-1 neurons in the hindbrain are activated through physiological mechanisms—or they can be activated through chemogenetics, optogenetics, things like that—you do get decrease in food intake, you get increase in avoidance behavior, you get stress responses," she said. "The drugs are activating that system differently. They're jumping over the neurons themselves and then directly accessing just a subset of the receptors."

Hayes followed up by asking Rinaman whether, if one could activate the endogenous GLP-1 system through a different therapeutic modality in addition to treating the system with a GLP-1R agonist, there would be a further enhancement of weight loss. Rinaman answered yes, citing research that demonstrated additional suppression of food intake when semaglutide was combined with chemogenetic activation of the GLP-1 neurons (Brierley et al., 2021). That might offer a good target for future pharmacotherapies, she suggested.

Penetrance of the Blood–Brain Barrier

Christian Hölscher, cofounder and chief scientific officer of Kariya Pharmaceuticals and a professor of neuroscience at the Henan University of Chinese Medicine, asked Drucker about the data that showed that tirzepatide and semaglutide have no effect in the mouse model of Alzheimer's disease. Perhaps the reason is that those drugs do not cross the blood–brain barrier, Hölscher suggested. Earlier GLP-1R agonists could cross into the brain and do have effects on the mouse model of Alzheimer's disease, but the newer drugs have been designed to stay in the blood for a very long time and do not really cross into the brain, said Hölscher.

Drucker agreed that these newer drugs do not meaningfully penetrate the brain, but Secher, Rinaman, and others have shown they do meaningfully signal to many regions deep within the brain. Furthermore, he continued, they produce 15 to 20 percent weight loss, which is mediated by many circuits in the brain. Given that, Drucker said, the key questions are, "Where do we need to go to activate the critical regions to achieve meaningful neuroprotection? And how might that differ from what we can activate peripherally with these medicines to produce powerful weight loss?" Perhaps, he suggested, GLP-1R agonists that get into the brain more efficiently might produce more neuroprotection, but would they also lead to more adverse events? A key question that remains to be answered is which drugs and which brain targets will maximize the neuroprotective benefits while minimizing adverse events.

Another workshop participant inquired about data that speak to differences in the nonlipidated versus lipidated GLP-1R agonists and their differential effects on blood–brain barrier penetrance. Secher said that to their surprise, her team has found that nonlipidated molecules penetrate the same way or show up in the same areas as lipidated molecules. "It's probably something more around this GLP-1 receptor recognition," she said.

Sex and Age Differences

Alexandra Sinclair, a professor of neurology at the University of Birmingham, asked whether there are sex or age differences in the distribution of the GLP-1 receptors around the brain or in the access of the GLP-1 receptor agonists into the brain. Secher answered that she has not systematically looked at sex differences in her mouse model but added that she should do that. Concerning aging, she said, there may well be some differences in the blood–brain barrier between young mice and very old mice, but she is not sure they could be detected with the methods she currently uses.

Rinaman said that unpublished data from her lab show that diet exposure during the perinatal period of development in rats can profoundly affect the axonal projections of the GLP-1 neurons, and it also seems to affect the expression of the receptors. Her lab is now studying whether those effects persist into adulthood. "I'm really excited about that because it suggests the potential for individual differences in the central GLP-1 system that could be attributed to dietary effects or perhaps stress exposures early in development," she said. This could help explain individual differences among humans in responsiveness to these drugs, including some well-known sex differences. For example, previous research has shown that females appear to be more sensitive to the ability of GLP-1R agonists to suppress food intake and body weight (e.g., Richard et al., 2016).

Hayes added that his lab has a paper under review looking at sex differences in response to GLP-1R agonists and how the estrous cycle affects the expression of the GCG gene, which codes for preproglucagon, and the GLP-1 receptor gene. When the GLP-1R agonists are administered during the estrous cycle affects how effective the drugs are in terms of weight loss. This could point to differing effects in human patients, for instance, between pre- and postmenopausal women, said Hayes.

GLP-1R Antagonists

Iván Montoya, director of the Division of Therapeutics and Medical Consequences at the National Institute on Drug Abuse (NIDA), asked about the effects of GLP-1R antagonists. Drucker said that there has been a series of attempts over time to develop these antagonists for the treatment of postbariatric hypoglycemia and other orphan conditions as well. "We don't have a lot of human data with prolonged exposure, other than in the context of hypoglycemia, that people have looked at," he said, so it is not clear what other effects, either beneficial or adverse, the antagonists might have. However, Drucker added, in the bariatric surgery hypoglycemia trials, there do not seem to be any adverse effects. "It's a question that would merit further study," he said.

Heterogeneity of Response

Fatima Cody Stanford, an associate professor of medicine and pediatrics and obesity medicine physician-scientist at the Massachusetts General Hospital and Harvard Medical School, said that as someone who has treated more than 3,000 patients with obesity, she does have strong data supporting the heterogeneity of response to GLP-1R agonists in practice. Some patients are nonresponders to the drugs, while others have a high response, and these distinct responses arise even within individual families. Ultimately, the only way she knows how well a patient will respond to the drug is to wait and see.

Hayes asked whether the GLP-1 receptors develop a tolerance similar to what is seen with opioid receptors in the brain. Drucker answered that it does happen sometimes that a person responds initially but then stops responding and does not achieve the desired weight loss. "Sometimes we switch them from one medicine to another, and sometimes people respond better, and other times they don't," he said. However, Drucker added, we just don't have enough data to know with any certainty what is going on at the receptor level or postreceptor level that is behind this phenomenon.

In sum, much current research is aimed at understanding the endogenous GLP-1 system in the brain, particularly how GLP-1R agonists gain access to certain regions of the brain and their effects once they are in the brain, but the complexity of GLP-1 pathways has so far kept scientists from developing a complete understanding of the system.

3

Learning from Those with Lived Experiences

HIGHLIGHTS

- Obesity is a medical condition involving multiple complex factors and is not related to self-discipline. (Nece)
- The new class of GLP-1R agonists can help in the treatment of binge eating, although their side effects and effectiveness may vary among individuals. (Nece)
- GLP-1R agonists can be very effective in helping people lose weight, but because of high demand they can sometimes be difficult to get. (Glanz, Nece)
- Even with a doctor's prescription and insurance coverage approval, some people have found it difficult to gain access to GLP-1R agonists. (Glanz)

NOTE: This list is the rapporteurs' summary of points made by the individual speakers identified, and the statements have not been endorsed or verified by the National Academies of Sciences, Engineering, and Medicine. They are not intended to reflect a consensus among workshop participants.

Lived experiences personalize the benefits and risks involved with the use of glucagon-like peptide 1 receptor (GLP-1R) agonists, said Kimberlei Richardson, an associate professor in the Department of Pharmacology at the Howard University College of Medicine. Two individuals with direct experience with GLP-1R agonists shared their perspectives. They spoke about the stigma that people with obesity or neurological disorders often face, their struggles to find effective treatments, and their experiences with the new GLP-1R agonists.

AN EXPERIENCE WITH BINGE EATING DISORDER AND OBESITY

Patricia Nece, a member of the National Academies Roundtable on Obesity Solutions[1] and the immediate past chair of the Obesity Action Coalition, spoke about her experiences with binge eating disorder and obesity. "I've had obesity since childhood," she said. "I don't remember a time when I wasn't one of the biggest people in the room. That, of course, exposed me to bullying, bias, stigma, and discrimination." And the effects of that stigma and bias are incredibly harmful.

She was always a very active kid, Nece said. She was on swim teams—including a synchronized swim team in college—rode a 10-speed bicycle for transportation and did gymnastics. "I was always very active, yet my weight was always high," she said. And although she found success in other areas of her life, including her professional and family life, she could never control her weight despite trying multiple diets. "I would lose some weight, and it would come back. I'd lose weight again on a different diet, and it would come back, usually bringing a few friendly extra pounds with it." As a result, she blamed herself for not being able to maintain the weight loss, she said, because that is what she consistently heard from medical professionals, the media, family, friends, and society in general.

It was only when she was in her 50s and started working with an obesity medicine specialist that she realized that obesity is a disease involving complex factors. At that point she had lost 120 pounds by pairing medical treatment with psychological treatment aimed at helping her cope with the weight bias that she had internalized and to reduce the stigma she felt. She also discovered that she had binge eating disorder. The binges had always been part of her life, she said, but she "didn't really see them as different or something that maybe I could seek treatment for."

Still, after Nece had lost the 120 pounds, she had difficulty maintaining the lower weight, and she started to regain some of it. That led her to start taking medication. She began with lorcaserin, marketed as Belviq, which helped her maintain the weight loss, though she did not lose much more. What it did help with, Nece said, was what she called the "food noise"[2] in her brain, the way she talked to herself about food. However, the drug's

---

[1] For more information on the Roundtable on Obesity Solutions, see https://www.national academies.org/our-work/roundtable-on-obesity-solutions (accessed November 11, 2024).

[2] *Food noise* refers to the intrusive thoughts about eating and food that can make it difficult for some people trying to lose weight to resist eating food that is not part of their diet.

manufacturer pulled it from the market in February 2020 at the request of the FDA because an increased risk of cancer had been observed in people taking it.

During the COVID-19 pandemic, Nece gained 50 pounds, which led her to decide, in consultation with her obesity medicine specialist, to try a GLP-1R agonist. She started with semaglutide, taking half of the normal starting dose for the treatment of diabetes. Unfortunately, it gave her severe intestinal and digestive problems, and her specialist told her that, judging from the experiences of his other patients, she would probably not adjust to those side effects. "The sad part was, I was pretty sure it was working," Nece said. "I can tell you exactly the place and time when my appetite returned."

It took her about 2 years before she was ready to try again, at which point she went with tirzepatide, which is a dual agonist for both GLP-1R and the glucose-dependent insulinotropic polypeptide (GIP) receptor. She was somewhat fatigued at the beginning and had a few gastrointestinal issues, but overall, Nece experienced few side effects, and she felt it was a successful drug for her. It helped with her binge eating disorder, in large part, she said, because it cut down on her normal food noise. Even when she drove past fast-food restaurants on her way to and from work, she no longer found herself thinking about food. The combination of psychological therapy and tirzepatide provided her with enough support that she could control her symptoms. And since Nece has started taking tirzepatide, she has lost about 20 percent of what she weighed at the time she began.

Despite the success that she and others have had with GLP-1R agonists, Nece said, a number of challenges remain, related to the effective prescribing and use of the drugs. One of the key challenges, she said, is training the people who prescribe them. In her experience, she said, doctors treating patients with obesity often write a prescription without providing any support for the patient or even offering any detailed instructions. She herself responded to tirzepatide by hardly eating at all. Fortunately, she continued, she had the resource of a nutritionist, who worked with her to develop a plan that combined her tirzepatide with an appropriate diet. However, most patients do not have that resource, she said, so training more providers in this area will be critical.

A second challenge, Nece said, is the silos that have been built between physical health and mental health. When discussing obesity with a patient, doctors rarely touch on psychological health, she said, but they should. She said this is particularly important for patients being put on GLP-1R agonists, since the drugs can lead to dramatic behavioral changes. In her case, she said, her entire approach to eating changed almost overnight from what she had known her whole life.

A SUCCESS STORY OF USING A GLP-1R AGONIST TO LOSE WEIGHT

Karen Glanz, George A. Weiss University Professor at the University of Pennsylvania Perelman School of Medicine and School of Nursing, spoke about her experiences using a GLP-1R agonist to lose weight, lower her cholesterol, and improve her liver function. She approached the topic as someone who has also conducted research in the field of obesity, nutrition, and activity for several decades (Glanz et al., 2005, 2006, 2021, 2023; Sallis and Glanz, 2009).

During that time and earlier years, she had her own struggles with weight, losing a substantial amount of weight, regaining it, losing it, and then regaining it. "This is a story that I think many people who are patients with these drugs have probably been through," she said, "and it's the biology as well as the behavior."

She had always followed a healthy eating lifestyle, and her interest in physical activity and her passion for an active lifestyle grew when she started triathlons. She loved the idea of physical activity as the way to a healthier body and mind, she continued, but she felt somewhat embarrassed to wear swimsuits and sports outfits that exposed more of her body. Despite this, Glanz said, she "continued [physical activity] with all the ups and downs of the weight."

Then, in 2023, Glanz's primary internist recommended that she should go on a statin, a cholesterol-lowering drug, for her high cholesterol. Glanz, frustrated with her weight struggles, asked about being prescribed a GLP-1 drug, specifically Wegovy, which her doctor did. But after getting the prescription and insurance authorization, the drug was not available. After a number of months of waiting, she found out from a colleague that if she switched from a commercial pharmacy to a university-based specialty pharmacy, she could get medication in a higher dose, so her doctor agreed to start her on Wegovy at 0.5 milligrams.

In nearly 11 months, she lost 46 pounds (Figure 3-1). Furthermore, her low-density lipoprotein (LDL) decreased significantly as she was taking both a statin and Wegovy, and her liver function tests returned to normal. "For me, this has been a miracle drug," she said.

DISCUSSION

Fatigue as a Side Effect of GLP-1R Agonists

Ellen Mowry, a workshop participant from Johns Hopkins University, asked Nece about the fatigue she reported experiencing when on GLP-1R

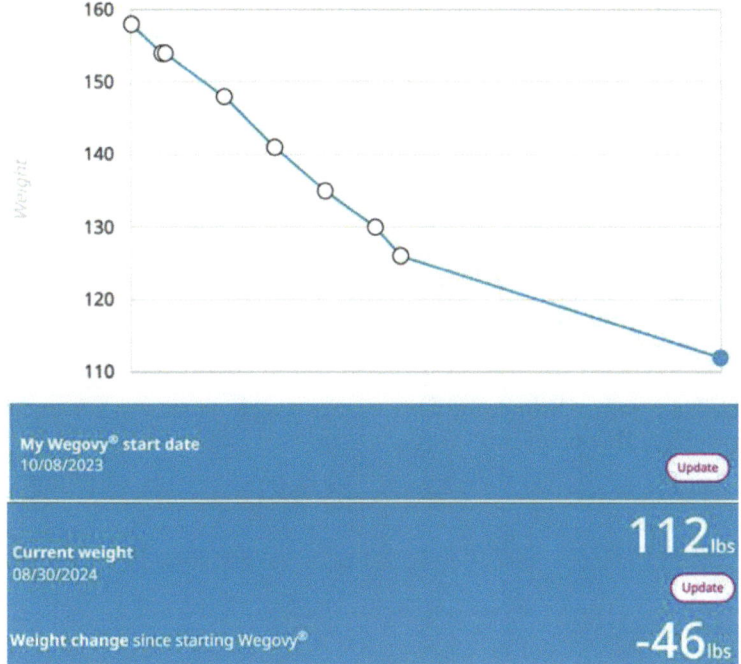

FIGURE 3-1 Personal weight loss on Wegovy.
SOURCE: Presented by Karen Glanz on September 10, 2024.

agonists. Nece said that on the day after she took the first dose of tirzepatide, she did not wake up until 1 p.m., when normally she had been waking up at 9:00 a.m., and she only woke up then because her doorbell rang. She did not feel fatigued while awake, she said, but she slept much more than usual. Now, after about a year of taking tirzepatide, the effect has gotten much better.

Jon Davis, a principal scientist at Novo Nordisk, added that researchers do not really understand the mechanism behind the sleepiness or fatigue caused by these drugs, but it would make sense that a tremendous reduction in appetite and caloric intake over a prolonged period of time could lead to fatigue. And Hayes commented that the typical satiety response includes sleep and rest, so the additional sleep that Nece experienced might be related to a satiating response. Finally, Patricia Sue Grigson, professor and chair of the Department of Neural and Behavioral Sciences at the Penn State College of Medicine, said that some of her rodent studies found that the rats had an increase in non-REM sleep following treatment with liraglutide (Fang et al., 2023).

Decreasing the Stigma Associated with Using GLP-1R Agonists

In response to a question about ways to decrease the stigma surrounding usage of the GLP-1R agonist, Nece said that weight bias, stigma, and discrimination are ubiquitous in society and that every individual can help make a difference. "I think the way to attack stigma with these medications is for everybody to start understanding what weight stigma is and speaking out about it," she said. She urged the members of the audience to start by examining their own internal biases. "The next time you're seeing somebody my size walking down the street, start noticing what are your automatic assumptions about that person. If you saw me, would you think I was even interested in weight management? You might not, but yet here I am." The next step is for people to speak out whenever they witness weight stigma, Nece said. "I think until we reduce weight stigma in society, we're going to have this problem."

4

Ingestive Behavior Disorders

HIGHLIGHTS

- Eating disorders are behavioral illnesses, not a matter of lifestyle choice. (Richardson)
- Preclinical and clinical evidence indicate that GLP-1R agonists could be an effective treatment for binge eating disorder and perhaps other eating disorders. (McElroy, Mietlicki-Baase, Richardson)
- GLP-1R agonists affect the behavior of dopamine neurons in the brain's reward regions, but the precise mechanisms remain unclear. Understanding them better could lead to insights into how GLP-1R agonists affect ingestive behavior disorders, such as binge eating. (Davis)
- One of the challenges for understanding the biological processes and changes in the GLP-1 signaling in the context of eating disorders is a shortage of funding opportunities for basic science or mechanistic studies in this area. (Mietlicki-Baase)

NOTE: This list is the rapporteurs' summary of points made by the individual speakers identified, and the statements have not been endorsed or verified by the National Academies of Sciences, Engineering, and Medicine. They are not intended to reflect a consensus among workshop participants.

Kimberlei Richardson said there is a common misconception that eating disorders are a matter of lifestyle choice, but, according to both the American Psychiatric Association and the National Institute of Mental Health, eating disorders are behavioral illnesses characterized by severe and persistent disturbance in eating behaviors and associated with distressing thoughts and emotions. The most common eating disorders are anorexia nervosa, bulimia nervosa, and binge eating disorder, she said, and approximately 9 percent of Americans, or 28.8 million people today, will have an eating disorder in their lifetime, and some 10,200 Americans die each year as a direct result of an eating disorder (Deloitte Access Economics, 2020). An estimated 42–52 percent of individuals diagnosed with binge eating disorder have a reported comorbidity of obesity, which increases the risk of mortality (Agüera et al., 2021; Udo and Grilo, 2018; Villarejo et al., 2012).

Significant evidence has been accumulated that GLP-1R agonists may be effective in treating such ingestive behavior disorders, Richardson said. For instance, a number of preclinical studies have indicated that these agonists play a role in regulating feeding and binge eating behaviors (Barrera et al., 2011; Holt et al., 2019; Mietlicki-Baase et al., 2013; Yamaguchi et al., 2017). There have also been clinical studies investigating the effect of GLP-1R agonists on binge eating behavior. In one, individuals treated with liraglutide demonstrated reduced binge eating behavior and lost more weight than those not treated with the drug (Robert et al., 2015). In another, GLP-1R agonists showed promising results in treating binge-eating behavior, though more rigorous clinical trials will be needed (Aoun et al., 2024).

Richardson concluded by listing the session objectives: (1) to review current knowledge about the mechanism of action of GLP-1R agonists and their therapeutic applications in ingestive behaviors, (2) to discuss the available scientific evidence of the clinical efficacy of these drugs for treating eating disorders, (3) to discuss the clinical consequences and adverse effects related to the use of GLP-1R agonists, and (4) to identify unique gaps and challenges in the field and provide suggestions for future research.

GLP-1R AGONISTS AND EATING DISORDERS

Susan L. McElroy, chief research officer at the Lindner Center of HOPE and Linda and Harry Fath Endowed Professor of Psychiatry and Behavioral Neuroscience at the University of Cincinnati College of Medicine, reviewed clinical evidence concerning the effectiveness of GLP-1R agonists in treating various eating disorders.

She began by listing all the feeding and eating disorders in the *Diagnostic and Statistical Manual of Mental Disorders*, 5th edition. The most common eating disorder is binge eating disorder, she said, and it is strongly associated with obesity. Bulimia nervosa is also associated with obesity, as is atypical anorexia nervosa, where people have all the psychological symptoms of anorexia but are normal weight, overweight, or obese.

There are also several disorders not listed in *Diagnostic and Statistical Manual of Mental Disorders* that are associated with obesity but that researchers really need to learn more about, she added. These include food addiction, which has a strong overlap with binge eating disorder, antipsychotic-induced binge eating, and hyperphagia and polyphagia, which are types of intense overeating observed with monogenetic obesity, that is, obesity caused by a mutation in a single gene.

Of all of these, she said, binge eating disorder has been the focus of the most scientific research. A number of drugs have been used in clinical trials to treat binge eating disorder. Four of them are on the market—bupropion-naltrexone, liraglutide, orlistat, and phentermine-topiramate—but none of these four have clear evidence of effectiveness in treating binge eating. Orlistat, for example, has shown positive results for weight loss but mixed results for binge eating (McElroy et al., 2012).

At least two studies have focused on the effects of liraglutide in people with binge eating and who are overweight. In one, 44 patients were randomly assigned to liraglutide or treatment as usual. According to the Binge Eating Scale, a self-report measure of binge eating symptomatology, there was a significant reduction in binge eating in both groups. However, only the liraglutide group showed a significant weight loss and reduction in body mass index (Robert et al., 2015).

The only randomized controlled trial of liraglutide for the treatment of binge eating disorder that McElroy was aware of was a small pilot study with 27 individuals who were given either liraglutide or a placebo for 17 weeks (Allison et al., 2022). Again, only the liraglutide group showed weight loss, while both groups had a reduction in the number of binge eating episodes per week over the course of the experiment.

The reduction in binge eating in the control groups of the two experiments was not unusual, McElroy said, as researchers regularly see a placebo response in binge eating disorder, and they have now identified ways to conduct clinical trials to minimize that. Given the small numbers of participants and the existence of a placebo effect, both studies have limitations, she said, but they do suggest that liraglutide reduces binge eating in addition to reducing weight. Furthermore, the drug has been shown to be safe, making it a good candidate for treating binge eating, she added.

Finally, McElroy described a study that her group carried out in patients with stable bipolar disorder and obesity. Many mental illnesses are associated with obesity, including bipolar disorder, she noted, so such studies are important. It was a 40-week, double-blind, placebo-controlled study, and the majority of these patients were on antipsychotics. Despite that, the patients given liraglutide had a marked decrease in weight (McElroy et al., 2024). Her team also carefully evaluated the patients for psychiatric side effects, including suicidality using the Columbia suicide scale,[1] and found no indication that liraglutide increased suicidality or caused mood instability—a concern with several other weight loss drugs. In addition, the team assessed binge eating behavior using the Binge Eating Scale and found that liraglutide significantly reduced binge eating behavior while also reducing hunger.

Finally, she said that her team prescribes GLP-1R agonists to some patients diagnosed with obesity and an eating disorder. They believe that there are preliminary data to suggest these compounds may be helpful in treating binge eating disorder, including binge eating disorder induced by antipsychotic medication and binge eating disorder in people who are of normal weight. They also believe that the compounds might be helpful for some people with bulimia nervosa, especially those who also have obesity. She warned, however, that GLP-1R agonists could be misused by people with anorexia nervosa in their efforts to lose weight.

McElroy said that when people with obesity come to her center for treatment, the clinicians evaluate them very carefully for eating disorders as well as other psychiatric disorders. "There is no doubt obesity and psychiatric disorders are related," she concluded, "and I think that's been a completely ignored area."

THE RESPONSE OF THE BRAIN'S REWARD REGIONS TO GLP-1R AGONISTS

Jon Davis spoke about research on how GLP-1R agonists affect dopaminergic neurons in the central nervous system, which are intimately involved with reward-seeking behavior.

He began by reviewing some clinical data from Novo Nordisk's STEP (Semaglutide Treatment Effect in People with Obesity) trial. Patients treated with 2.4 milligrams of semaglutide lost an average of about 16 percent of their body weight over 60 weeks, although there was a plateau around 52 weeks after which they lost little more weight. Then, after patients were removed from the drug, they regained an average of about 10 percent of their original body weight over the next 60 weeks, leaving them at about 6 percent down from their weight at the beginning of the trial (Wilding et al., 2022).

---

[1] "The Columbia Suicide Severity Rating Scale (C-SSRS) is a short questionnaire that can be administered quickly in the field by responders with no formal mental health training, and it is relevant in a wide range of settings and for individuals of all ages." https://www.samhsa.gov/resource/dbhis/columbia-suicide-severity-rating-scale-c-ssrs (accessed November 10, 2024).

Given these results, Davis said, researchers at Novo Nordisk were interested in what leads to the plateau in weight loss and what leads to the weight regain once patients stop taking semaglutide. One interesting result, he added, related to how long-term use of a GLP-1R agonist affects the reward regions in the CNS. Novo Nordisk scientists gave patients a 3-milligram dose of liraglutide—the highest dose approved for weight loss—for 35 weeks and examined their brains' response to palatable food cues. What they found was that reward regions in the orbital frontal cortex, when corrected for body mass index, responded more strongly to the food cues after the 35 weeks of liraglutide than they had before. These were patients who had lost a significant amount of weight, he said, but their brains' reward regions were reacting more strongly than before. "This would not be what we would predict," he said, as patients who have been treated for many months with a GLP-1R agonist generally report having less appetite and interest in food.

To explore potential mechanisms, the researchers took a closer look at the response of the brain's reward regions—particularly its dopamine system—to GLP-1R agonists. He showed a diagram of the brain's mesolimbic dopamine system, with a specific focus on the ventral tegmental area (VTA) and its projections to the nucleus accumbens as well as to the frontal cortex (see Figure 4-1). Over the past 50 to 60 years, Davis said, this system has been intensely studied for its ability to regulate substance use disorder as well as reward-based learning and reinforcement learning, but in the past 20 years it has become clear that this process controls appetite as well. And it turns out that GLP-1R agonists and other incretins (gastrointestinal hormones that regulate insulin secretion) modulate this mesolimbic dopamine system. Generally speaking, Davis explained, things that increase dopamine

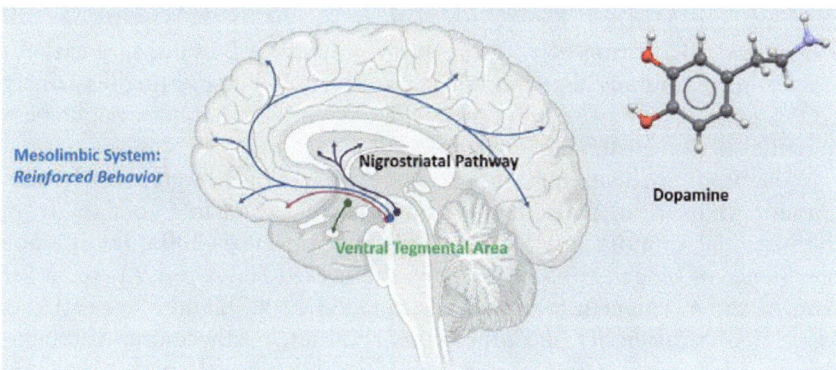

FIGURE 4-1 The CNS mesolimbic dopamine system.
NOTE: CNS = central nervous system.
SOURCE: Presented by Jon Davis on September 10, 2024.

levels motivate behaviors, while things that decrease dopamine levels do the opposite.

So how do GLP-1R agonists affect dopamine levels in this system? In one study that examined this issue, researchers administered exendin-4, a GLP-1 agonist, directly into the lateral ventricle of rats to see what happened to the activity of dopamine neurons in the VTA. The key result, Davis said, is that when the drug was administered, it not only reduced anticipation and consumption of palatable foods in the rats, but it also decreased the activity of dopamine neurons (Konanur et al., 2020). One might assume, then, that triggering GLP-1 receptors in the rodent brain has its effect on appetite and body weight by reducing the activity of dopamine neurons, he said. However, it is not that simple, as a similar study had very different results. In that study, mice were given semaglutide in their abdominal cavity, and its effects on appetite and dopamine signaling in the VTA were studied. Again, the animals showed decreased appetite and lost weight, but there was an increase in the activity of dopamine neurons (Kooij et al., 2024).

The differences between the two studies could be the dose used or the particular GLP-1R agonist that was administered, Davis said. It could also be the method of administration, either directly into the CNS or in the periphery, which would involve crossing the blood–brain barrier. "It is not clear at this point actually what's going on with how these drugs are activating or engaging with the dopamine system," he said.

Thus, he concluded, more studies are needed clarify exactly how the brain monoamine system is affected by GLP-1R agonists.

BINGE EATING AND THE ENDOGENOUS GLP-1 SYSTEM

Elizabeth Mietlicki-Baase, associate professor in the Department of Exercise and Nutrition Sciences at the University of Buffalo, spoke about studies in lab animals aimed at understanding how binge eating may affect GLP-1 expression in the brain and whether GLP-1R agonists might be a potential treatment for binge eating.

She began by defining binge eating as consuming a larger than normal amount of food in a discrete period of time. According to data from the National Comorbidity Survey Replication in 2001–2003, the lifetime prevalence of binge eating behavior in the United States is 4.9 percent for women and 4.0 percent for men (Hudson et al., 2007), and binge eating is associated with obesity and other comorbidities. Furthermore, Mietlicki-Baase added, binge eating is not limited to those people with diagnosed eating disorder. "Plenty of people might binge eat," she said. "It just doesn't reach clinical diagnosis level. So, this is a problem that affects a lot of people."

The current treatment options for binge eating disorder are limited, she said. They include evidence-based psychological treatments such as cognitive behavioral therapy; lisdexamfetamine, which is a psychostimulant drug approved by the FDA for the treatment of binge eating disorder; and some off-label uses of pharmacotherapies. Given those limited options, Mietlicki-Baase became interested in GLP-1 as a pharmacological target that might point to a more effective treatment of the disorder (Balantekin et al., 2024; McElroy et al., 2018).

She and her team focused their attention on the nucleus of the solitary tract (NST), which produces preproglucagon, the precursor to GLP-1, and which has direct projections to many areas of the brain—particularly areas relevant to food intake and food reward. Therefore, they hypothesized that binge eating in laboratory animals would lead to changes in GLP-1 expression in the hindbrain.

Binge eating is modeled in rodents by limiting the animals' access to a particularly palatable food, such as vegetable shortening, so that they eat more of it than if they were given more regular access. Control animals might be given access to the palatable food for 1 hour every day, for instance, while the trial animals might get access for 1 hour on every other day. When those trial animals do get their access, they overeat, or "binge." (The animals are all given as much water and regular rat chow as they want.) This is not the same as binge eating in humans, Mietlicki-Baase noted, since it is missing the various psychological aspects and cognitive aspects to the disorder that are present in people. But the overeating aspect is similar, and this intermittent provision of palatable foods is a standard model for binge eating in rats. Mietlicki-Baase referred to what the rats do as "binge-like eating" to acknowledge the differences.

Her group's first study looked at whether binge-like eating affected GLP-1 expression in the NST of male rats. Some rats were given intermittent access to the palatable food, while the control group had regular access. After nine weeks, they collected tissue and blood samples from the animals and performed various measurements. There were no differences in body weight between the two groups, which was critical, she noted, because it let them look at the questions about central and peripheral GLP-1 in the absence of body weight changes that could act as a confounding factor.

Examining GLP-1 receptor expression in the NST, the researchers found no differences between the two groups of rats. However, the expression of the GLP-1 precursor, preproglucagon, in the NST was quite different, being drastically reduced in the rats with only intermittent access to feeding (Mukherjee et al., 2020). Her group interpreted this as the rats' losing a signal that tells them to stop eating.

Interestingly, plasma GLP-1 was actually increased in the rats with intermittent access. Her group was puzzled by this, but they now think it could be due to the rats anticipating the food. There is some evidence in the literature, she said, that rats on a scheduled access of feeding have anticipatory increases in circulating GLP-1.

Given the changes in the NST triggered by binge eating, Mietlicki-Baase wondered what other parts of the brain might be involved. They looked at the VTA, which Davis had described in the previous presentation as being an important part of the brain's reward system. They found that, interestingly, GLP-1 receptor expression was increased in the VTA in the rats that had "binged." Given that there seem to be various effects of binge-like eating on the GLP-1 system, she said, "we're very interested in understanding whether increasing central GLP-1 signaling could be a strategy to ameliorate binge eating."

To see whether there might be sex differences in how binge-like eating affects the GLP-1 system, Mietlicki-Baase's group carried out a similar experiment on female rats. In this case they saw no difference between the intermittent access group and the control group in the expression of the preproglucagon in the NST, but they did see greater GLP-1 receptor expression in the NST in animals with free access to palatable food compared with a chow-only control group. There were no differences in plasma GLP-1 among the groups.

In terms of future directions and challenges in the area, Mietlicki-Baase highlighted several points. Given the differences they saw between males and females, her lab would like to further explore potential sex differences in binge eating and GLP-1. Furthermore, she added, "There is really a need to understand some of these key biological processes and changes in GLP-1 signaling in the context of binge eating and what the timing of these effects is. We did these studies after about 8 weeks of binge eating. We don't know what happens earlier."

Finally, she wishes to investigate the potential effects of other hormonal systems. "We know with the advent of dual- and tri-agonists and other hormonal systems being targeted for obesity treatment, there could be a more effective drug or combination therapy that we have yet to investigate," she said.

As for challenges, she said that finding funding for further basic science research to understand the neurobiology of eating disorders is one of the biggest.

DISCUSSION

The Effect of GLP-1R on Dopamine

Brian Fiske asked if there have been any preclinical data on how GLP-1R agonists affect dopamine specifically in the context of motor control, which is important information for neurodegenerative diseases as Parkinson's disease. Davis said he was not aware of research looking at phasic firing of the dopamine neurons and locomotion or other neurodegenerative-like endpoints. What has been done so far, he said, has focused just on appetite, food intake, and body weight endpoints.

In response to an online question about whether anyone has looked at the effects of GLP-1R agonists on dopaminergic neurons in the VTA in terms of slice preparations, Davis answered that Matthew Hayes and his lab have done a lot of work on that and have found that GLP-1 activity usually dampens the activity of the dopamine system. However, a recent report observed that administering semaglutide increased VTA dopamine signaling during reward collection (Kooij et al., 2024). "If you think about what would be clinically efficacious for safe body weight loss," he said, "increasing dopamine might be the best way to go, so you don't have to worry about anhedonia, you don't have to worry about suicidal ideations." Particularly, in the case of the FDA-approved anti-obesity drug bupropion-naltrexone, the reported mechanism of action is blocking dopamine transport, leading to more dopamine in the synapse. This does seem to indicate that increasing dopamine may be a safe and effective way to lower body weight, concluded Davis.

The Potential Benefits of Co-Agonists

Richardson asked Mietlicki-Baase for her thoughts on co-agonism—that is, the combining of two agonists—in the treatment of binge eating. Mietlicki-Baase began by speaking about the hurdles in getting funding for studies testing co-agonism strategies to reduce binge eating. "Especially the basic science mechanistic studies can be a challenge to find agencies that are willing to support that research," she said regarding investigation of binge eating. "I think that that may improve as these dual- and tri-agonists and next generation drugs are shown to be effective in obesity treatment." And, she continued, it is possible that the repurposing of dual- and tri-agonists toward binge eating disorder or bulimia nervosa might become a more attractive area of research to fund as more evidence appears. In particular, she pointed to amylin[2] in combination with GLP-1R agonists such as semaglutide as having great promise in treating obesity and other disorders. Some preclinical work has been done to understand the role of amylin in binge eating, she said, and amylin seems to be affected in models of intermittent food access, but much more research needs to be done

---

[2] Amylin is a peptide hormone secreted along with insulin from the beta cells in the pancreas. It plays a role in regulating both blood sugar and satiety.

before it will be possible to turn this work into a pharmaceutical treatment for binge eating.

Davis added that a great deal of preclinical work indicates that amylin is probably a stronger suppressor of palatable food intake than other GLP-1R agonists, so amylin is a good molecule to be looking at for treatment of binge eating. More generally, he said that as more work is done with dual- and tri-agonists, he expects that there will be a greater focus on various obesity-related complications such as anxiety, depression, and binge eating, since the treatments will have the potential to address more than just obesity.

In sum, many workshop participants have shown that not only are GLP-1R agonists effective in treating obesity, but they have also shown promise against other eating disorders such as binge eating. Their effect on eating disorders seems to be at least partially dependent on their actions on dopamine neurons in the brain's reward regions, though much more research is needed to understand exactly how they work.

5

Substance Use Disorder and Alcohol Use Disorder

HIGHLIGHTS

- Preclinical and clinical evidence shows that GLP-1R agonists act to decrease drug use and seeking for a wide variety of substances including alcohol, nicotine, and opioids. (Farokhnia, Grigson, Jerlhag, Schmidt, Xu)
- GLP-1R agonists reduce alcohol consumption in rats, and a major reason for that effect seems to be that the agonists act on the brain's dopamine system to block the rewarding properties of alcohol. (Jerlhag)
- Unlike GLP-1R agonists, DPP-4 inhibitors do not seem to have any effect on alcohol use, even though their action in the body is to increase the amount of GLP-1. (Farokhnia)
- The GLP-1R agonist exendin-4 has been shown to decrease drug-seeking behavior during withdrawal in rats that previously self-administered cocaine. (Schmidt)
- Exendin-4 seems to have its suppressive effect on drug seeking in rats at least in part by activating inhibitory GABA neurons, which in turn suppress dopamine cell activity in the VTA. (Schmidt)
- A small-scale clinical trial found that a GLP-1R agonist was effective in reducing craving for opioids among people with opioid use disorder. (Grigson)

continued

- Trial emulations using real-world data indicate that semaglutide is effective against a number of substance use disorders, including alcohol use disorder, cannabis use disorder, tobacco use disorder, and opioid overdose risk. (Xu)

NOTE: This list is the rapporteurs' summary of points made by the individual speakers identified, and the statements have not been endorsed or verified by the National Academies of Sciences, Engineering, and Medicine. They are not intended to reflect a consensus among workshop participants.

Lorenzo Leggio, clinical director and deputy scientific director at the National Institute on Drug Abuse (NIDA) and current Chief of the Clinical Psychoneuroendocrinology and Neuropsychopharmacology Section, a joint NIDA and National Institute on Alcohol Abuse and Alcoholism (NIAAA) laboratory at the National Institutes of Health (NIH) Intramural Research Program, provided information on the numbers of "deaths of despair" in the United States from 1900 to 2017. These are deaths due to suicide, drugs, alcohol, and alcohol-related diseases such as liver disease. "Every 4.5 minutes, someone is dying in the United States because of addiction," Leggio said.

Unfortunately, he said, there is still a misconception that alcohol and substance use disorder are no more than "bad behaviors" or a personal choice, but there are clear scientific data showing that addiction is a brain disease (Heilig et al., 2021; Leshner, 1997; Volkow et al., 2016). Furthermore, he added, there are treatments that can help patients. There are effective behavioral treatments, and there are also medications approved by the FDA for treating opioid, tobacco, and alcohol use disorders, although still more medications are needed, he added.

The search for new medications has been aided by the recognition that the interplay and the connections between the brain and the body, including the heart–brain axis and the gut–brain axis are very important in addiction. Glucagon-like peptide-1, or GLP-1, is a key element in the gut–brain axis, he said, and the question has been raised whether the GLP-1 system might be a new target for treating addictions. There have been a number of anecdotal reports of people on GLP-1 receptor (GLP-1R) agonists experiencing reduced cravings for alcohol, tobacco, and drugs (Doucleff, 2023; Tirrell, 2023), Leggio said, "and as a physician, I really think it's very important to listen to these people."

Scientists have been working to understand the role of the GLP-1 system in addiction, he said, and there is already a robust literature on the topic (for recent review, see Bruns et al., 2024). In this session, he continued, the speakers would discuss where the field stands in terms of scientific evidence on the use of GLP-1R agonists and related drugs in the treatment of addiction.

PRECLINICAL STUDIES EXAMINING THE EFFECTS OF GLP-1R AGONISTS ON ALCOHOL CONSUMPTION

Elisabet Jerlhag, a professor of pharmacology at the University of Gothenburg, Sweden, provided an overview of preclinical studies—primarily laboratory studies in rats—of the effects of GLP-1R agonists on alcohol consumption. As background, she noted that alcohol use disorder cannot be modeled in animals with a single model, so researchers use different models to reflect the different aspects of the disorder.

One common model is the intermittent access model, in which rats are given both water and alcohol to drink on every second day and have access only to water on the days in between. What happens in these situations in that the rats will quickly come to drink significant amounts of alcohol on the days that it is available, to the point that their blood alcohol levels correspond with intoxication in humans.

Jerlhag's group used this model to test the effect of various GLP-1R agonists on alcohol intake in rats (see Figure 5-1). An early study showed that exendin-4 reduced alcohol intake in a dose-dependent manner (Egecioglu et al., 2013), but in retrospect the effect was quite small, she said. Later studies found much larger reductions in alcohol intake with liraglutide (Vallöf et al., 2016) and with dulaglutide (Vallöf et al., 2020). The earlier studies were done in male rats, Jerlhag said, but when her group added female rats to their investigations, they found a similar decrease in alcohol intake (Vallöf et al., 2020). Also, she added, there were no indications that the rats were building a tolerance to the GLP-1R agonists, and in some cases—the males but not the females—the treatment effect persisted after the rats were no longer receiving the drugs. Yet another experiment found that semaglutide reduced alcohol intake in both male and female rats in a dose-dependent manner (Aranäs et al., 2023). A group at NIDA reported similar findings on semaglutide and alcohol intake that same year (Chuong et al., 2023).

To see where the GLP-1R agonists were acting in the brain, Jerlhag's group used fluorescently marked semaglutide, which they found in the nucleus accumbens in rats that were given alcohol but not in control animals (Aranäs et al., 2023). Thus, the possibility should be considered that alcohol drinking changes the penetration of the drug into the brain, she said.

A second model that the group used for alcohol use disorder was relapse drinking. In this model, the rats consume alcohol for about 3 months, it is

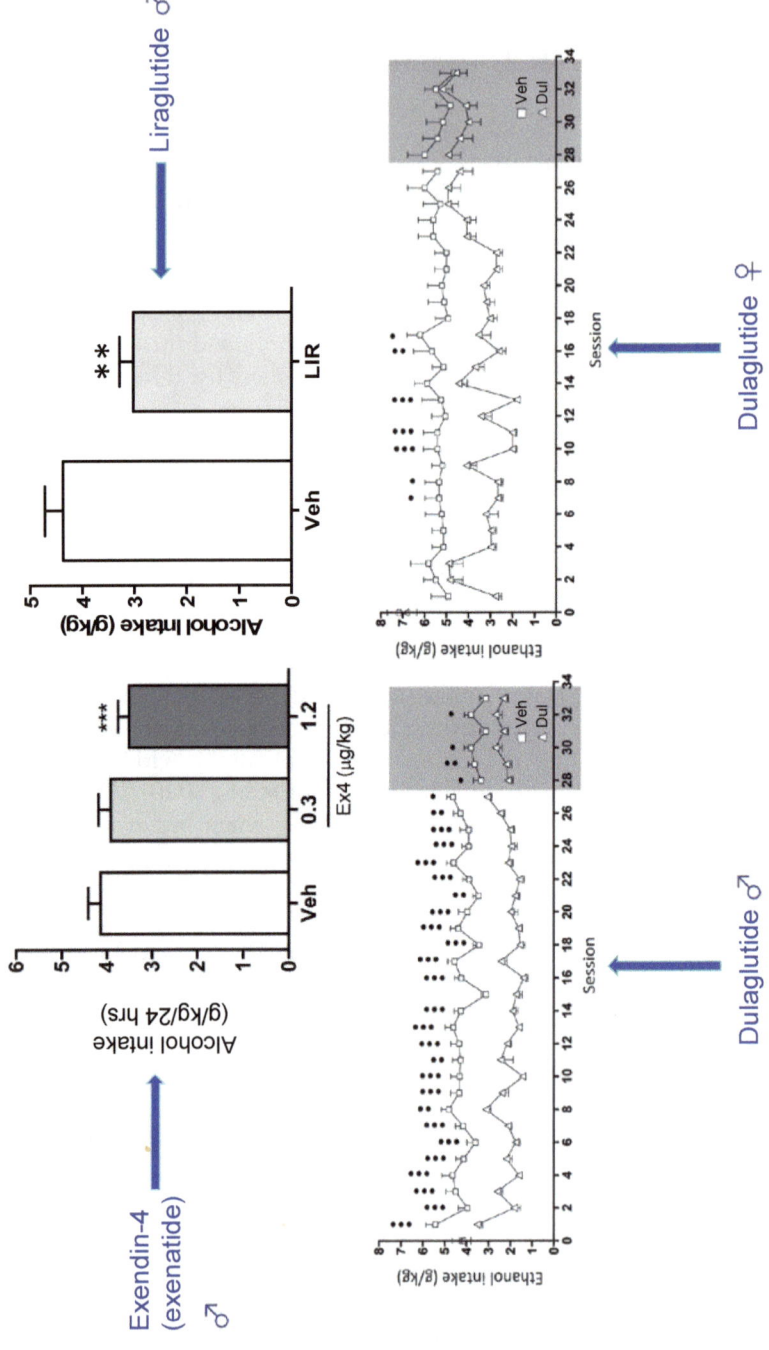

FIGURE 5-1 GLP-1R agonist reduces alcohol intake in rodents.
SOURCE: Presented by Elisabet Jerlhag on September 10, 2024. Adapted from Egecioglu et al., 2013; Vallöf et al., 2016, 2019.

taken away for 2 weeks, and then it is introduced again. In this situation the rats drink even more alcohol than they did before, which has been suggested as being parallel with alcohol craving in humans. Semaglutide was shown to prevent this relapse drinking in the rats (Aranäs et al., 2023). This is also observed by both exendin-4 and liraglutide, said Jerlhag.

A third model looked at the motivation to consume alcohol. In this case, rats are trained to press a lever to obtain alcohol, and their motivation is judged both by the total number of lever presses in a given period of time, such as 1 hour, and also by the "break point," which is the maximum number of times a rat will press the lever to get a single alcohol reward. By these measures, both exendin-4 and liraglutide reduced rats' motivation to consume alcohol (Egecioglu et al., 2013; Vallöf et al., 2016). In the case of liraglutide, that decrease in motivation persisted even after the rats stopped receiving the drug (Vallöf et al., 2016).

Jerlhag said that she believes the effects of these GLP-1R agonists on alcohol consumption have to do with the rewarding properties of alcohol. In both rats and humans, the desire to drink alcohol is driven to some extent by the rewards the brain associates with that drinking, and, indeed, in humans it has been shown that individuals who experience a great deal of reward from drinking alcohol are at a higher risk for alcohol use disorder later in life (King et al., 2021). In humans, the rewarding experience has been correlated to an increase in dopamine in the ventral striatum (Boileau et al., 2003), and this can also be seen in rodents. "So," Jerlhag said, "we can model something in animals that also is seen in humans. And we hypothesize that that reflects reward in rodents as it does in humans."

In experiments to test this, Jerlhag's team has found that while alcohol leads to a dopamine increase in rats' brains, treatment with exendin-4, liraglutide, or semaglutide blocks the effect (Aranäs et al., 2023; Egecioglu et al., 2013; Vallöf et al., 2016). So, they hypothesize that GLP-1 receptor agonists prevent a rat from feeling the usual reward it would get from alcohol, which contributes to a reduced alcohol intake, reduced motivation to drink alcohol, and prevention of relapse drinking.

These effects all take place in the brain. "Studies have shown that the brain GLP-1 receptors are quite important to regulate alcohol intake, but not the body GLP-1 receptors," Jerlhag said. And there are a number of specific brain areas that seem to be involved, including the nucleus accumbens, some parts of the ventral tegmental area (VTA), the nucleus of the solitary tract (NST), and the laterodorsal tegmental nucleus (LDTg), which is interconnected with the VTA.

Relatedly, Jerlhag mentioned that nicotine use has also been studied in lab animals, with GLP-1R agonists found to prevent nicotine-related behaviors. As with alcohol, dopamine release is prevented, and the motivation to consume nicotine is affected. Both exentin-4 and liraglutide have been shown to have these effects.

In closing, Jerlhag pointed to several next steps. She suggested, for instance, that future studies explore why different GLP-1R agonists have different outcomes. It would be useful to explore the mechanisms of action for these agonists in greater detail, and it would be valuable to study the reasons for the sex differences that are sometimes seen in response to the agonists.

DPP-4 INHIBITORS AND ALCOHOL CONSUMPTION IN RATS

Mehdi Farokhnia, a physician-scientist at NIH's intramural research program at NIDA and NIAAA, expanded on the preclinical work studying the effects of GLP-1R agonists on alcohol consumption by describing similar studies on the effects of dipeptidyl peptidase-4 (DPP-4) inhibitors on alcohol consumption in mice and rats. DPP-4 inhibitors, which are used to treat diabetes, act in the body by increasing the levels of GLP-1, which in turn inhibits glucagon production, increasing the secretion of insulin and decreasing the level of blood glucose. Since DPP-4 inhibitors increase GLP-1 levels, they are a natural candidate for treating alcohol or drug addiction.

Offering some background on DPP-4 inhibitors, Farokhnia said that GLP-1 has a very short half-life in the body because it is degraded by DPP-4. Thus DPP-4 inhibition is an alternative approach to GLP-1R agonists for stimulating the GLP-1 system by increasing the amount of GLP-1 circulated in the body.

Farokhnia's group initially tested the effects of two GLP-1R agonists, liraglutide and semaglutide, in male rats, and both reduced alcohol intake. Then, focusing more on semaglutide, they tested both male and female mice and rats across different paradigms, including binge-like drinking and dependence-associated drinking, and found that semaglutide reduced alcohol intake with no sex differences between males and females (Chuong et al., 2023).

To date, he noted, there has been only one clinical trial of a GLP-1R agonist in the treatment of alcohol use disorder. This was a 26-week, double-blind, placebo-controlled clinical trial of extended release exenatide (Klausen et al., 2022). There was no difference in the primary outcome—percentage of heavy drinking days—between the exenatide group and the placebo group. However, in a post hoc analysis, the researchers found that exenatide demonstrated a significant effect in reducing alcohol intake in those patients who had a body mass index (BMI) greater than 30. In further analyses using functional magnetic resonance imaging, they found that exenatide reduced cue reactivity (how the patients' brains responded when showed cues that would trigger thoughts about drinking), while positron emission tomography (PET) data showed that exenatide reduced dopamine transfer availability.

Given the preclinical work that GLP-1R agonists can reduce alcohol intake in rodents and the clinical work showing that they may have a similar effect in people, at least those with a high BMI, Farokhnia's team examined the possibility that DPP-4 inhibitors might also reduce alcohol intake. They have tested linagliptin, which does not cross the blood–brain barrier, and omarigliptin, which does. They used different paradigms, including drinking in the dark in mice, which is a model of binge-like drinking, and also a dependence-associated model of alcohol intake in rats. So far, though, they have seen no indication that DPP-4 inhibitors might reduce alcohol intake.

To examine the potential effectiveness of GLP-1R agonists and DPP-4 inhibitors in treating alcohol use disorders from a different angle, Farokhnia's group worked with electronic health records data from the Department of Veterans Affairs' Veterans Aging Cohort Study. In particular, they examined people who had been treated with GLP-1R agonists or DPP-4 inhibitors and compared them to those who had not been treated with either. To estimate how much the individuals in the study drank, the researchers relied on the Alcohol Use Disorders Identification Test–Consumption (AUDIT-C), which asks three questions on alcohol drinking. The researchers only included people with an AUDIT-C score greater than 0, indicating some level of drinking at baseline, and used various statistical techniques to try to make sure that each pair of groups being compared matched up well on all the variables beyond the treatment condition. One of the strengths of this unpublished study was its size, with well over 10,000 people included in each of the groups used in the comparisons.

Additionally, the researchers examined how the two groups differed in their change in alcohol use from the beginning of treatment to the end. They found that those who had been treated with GLP-1R agonists showed a greater reduction in drinking than those in the control group or the DPP-4 inhibitor recipients. When restricted to those with a diagnosis of alcohol use disorder or those who had an AUDIT-C score of at least 8 (indicating hazardous drinking), the difference was dramatically greater—those who were treated with GLP-1R agonists had a much greater decrease in AUDIT-C scores from baseline to follow-up, said Farokhnia.

Again, however, the DPP-4 inhibitors showed no effect on alcohol use, either in the comparison between DPP-4 inhibitor users and a control or in the comparison between DPP-4 inhibitor users and GLP-1R agonist users in the unpublished study. "I always say this is the only time I was very happy to see negative results," Farokhnia said, "because it replicates our preclinical findings." In short, he concluded, "both preclinically and clinically we see that GLP-1R agonists reduce alcohol intake, and DPP-4 inhibitors don't."

He closed by saying that his team is carrying out a clinical trial of semaglutide in people with alcohol use disorder whose results should be available in a few years, and a number of similar clinical trials are being conducted in the United States and Europe. The idea that GLP-1R agonists could be an effective treatment against alcohol use disorder has been getting a great deal of attention in the media (Doucleff, 2023; Johnson, 2024; Leslie, 2023; Resnick, 2024; Tirrell, 2023), but as he and a group of colleagues in the field argued in a commentary published a few months before the workshop (Leggio et al., 2023), it will be too early to make judgments about the efficacy of these drugs until the data from clinical trials begin to appear.

PRECLINICAL STUDIES ON THE USE OF GLP-1R AGONISTS TO DECREASE COCAINE USE

Heath D. Schmidt, director of the Laboratory of Neuropsychopharmacology at the University of Pennsylvania, spoke about experiments done with GLP-1R agonists in preclinical models of cocaine use disorder. One of his lab's goals is to identify novel anti-addiction therapies, and some of the agonists appear promising for that purpose.

The work in his lab uses the drug self-administration/reinstatement paradigm. Rats are implanted with jugular catheters, and after they have recovered from the surgery they are put into operant chambers where they can press a lever to get an intravenous infusion of cocaine. Typically, they allow the rats to self-administer cocaine for 21 days, at which point the cocaine solution is replaced with a saline solution for 5–7 days. During this abstinence period, the rats reduce their lever pressing. At this point the researchers can reinstate a rat's drug seeking—that is, get the rat to press the lever more often—by re-exposing the animal to the same stimuli that cause cocaine-addicted humans to relapse, such as giving it an acute injection of cocaine (Hernandez et al., 2018).

To test whether a GLP-1R agonist would decrease the rats' cocaine-seeking behavior, Schmidt's group pretreated rats with exendin-4 before they reintroduced the cocaine solution after 1 week of abstinence. While the control rats that had not been pretreated with exendin-4 pressed the lever repeatedly seeking the cocaine, the rats given exendin-4 pressed it much less often, and the rats given the highest dose of exendin-4 pressed the lever less than one-third as often as the control rats.

The group was excited about the findings, he said, because "as far as we knew, it was the first demonstration that a GLP-1 receptor agonist could reduce drug seeking in a reinstatement model." But they also wanted to determine whether the effect was due, at least in part, to activating GLP-1 receptors in the brain.

To see if the exendin-4 peptide penetrated the brain, the team put a fluorescent tag on the exendin-4 peptides and used that fluorescent tag to track the drug's distribution throughout the brain. They found that exendin-4 did cross the blood–brain barrier and that it ended up in nuclei that were known to regulate drug seeking, including the VTA, the nucleus accumbens, and the laterodorsal tegmental nucleus (Hernandez and Schmidt, 2019; Hernandez et al., 2018, 2021). Another study in Schmidt's lab, whose data have not yet been published, found that the exendin-4 induced c-Fos expression in the VTA, suggesting that it was activating neurons in the brain.

In another unpublished study, Schmidt's lab looked to see which cells in the midbrain were expressing GLP-1 receptors. They found that GLP-1R transcripts were primarily expressed in Gad1-positive neurons in the VTA. When they looked at dopamine neurons in the VTA, they found no expression of GLP-1 transcripts. "These findings indicate that GLP-1 receptors are primarily expressed in GABA neurons in the VTA," he said. The findings were confirmed by a second unpublished study that used single-nucleus RNA sequencing to look for GLP-1 receptor transcript expression in all cell types of the VTA.

These findings, Schmidt said, "support the hypothesis that the suppressive effects of exendin-4 in cocaine seeking may be due in part to activating inhibitory midbrain GABA neurons."

To examine what is going on at the cellular level in more detail, Schmidt's lab recently ran an in vivo fiber photometry experiment that allowed them to record intracellular calcium dynamics—specifically in GABA neurons of the VTA—during cocaine reinstatement tests. As before, the exendin-4 significantly reduced how often the rats pressed the lever during reinstatement tests, and they also found an increase in the activity of GABA neurons in only the exendin-4-treated rats when they were drug seeking. In a second experiment with similar technique, they looked at intracellular calcium dynamics in the dopamine neurons of the VTA rather than the GABA neurons. The control rats demonstrated a significant increase in dopamine cell activity associated with lever pressing, but this neuronal activity was not present in the rats pretreated with exendin-4.

These data point to the group's current working hypothesis about how exendin-4 reduces cocaine-seeking behavior in rats, Schmidt said. The GABA neurons act to inhibit the dopamine neurons. When the control rats are re-exposed to cocaine after the week of abstinence, they push the lever at a high rate—that is, they are more persistent in seeking the cocaine, and there is an increase in dopamine cell activity, while the inhibitory GABA neurons are relatively quiet. However, treatment with exendin-4 activates the rats' midbrain inhibitory GABA neurons, which in turn leads to decreased phasic dopamine cell firing and reduced drug seeking.

In summary, Schmidt said that systemic administration of a GLP-1R agonist, specifically exendin-4, attenuates drug seeking. The effective doses are well tolerated in cocaine-dependent rats; that is, they do not affect food intake, and they do not produce malaise-like effects. These preclinical findings support using GLP-1R agonists for treating cocaine use disorder. The data also suggest that the mechanism by which exendin-4 suppresses the drug-seeking behavior involves activating inhibitory GABA neurons.

Schmidt closed with a list of unanswered questions and future directions. A key research direction, he said, should be to determine the downstream molecular and cellular mechanisms underlying the efficacy of GLP-1R agonists on drug-seeking and drug-taking behaviors. Part of the research should involve disentangling the relative contributions of postsynaptic versus presynaptic receptors in the behavioral responses to these agonists. He also suggested that researchers explore whether they can target central GLP-1-producing circuits in the brain to selectively reduce drug-mediated behaviors, study which GLP-1R agonists are most effective in reducing drug- and alcohol-seeking behaviors and look for any adverse effects of GLP-1R agonists in humans with substance use disorders. As an example, Schmidt said, he is particularly concerned about the potential for adverse gastrointestinal effects in humans with opioid use disorder. Finally, he concluded, he would like research to address the question of whether approaches targeting GLP-1 and additional neuropeptide systems with overlapping functional activity would be more effective and better tolerated than treatments with a single GLP-1R agonist alone.

CLINICAL TRIALS OF GLP-1R AGONISTS FOR TREATING OPIOID USE DISORDER

Patricia Sue Grigson said that people in the field have long thought about substance use disorders—and opioid use disorder in particular—in terms of their hijacking reward pathways, but perhaps they should instead be thought about in terms of their hijacking "need pathways." "Why would individuals take such chances with their lives, with the lives of their offspring?" Grigson asked. Is it because they are seeking a reward or because they are desperately seeking to satisfy a need?

If addiction is hijacking substrates involved in these "need pathways," she asked, could opioid seeking and taking be reduced by treatment with a known satiety agent? She and her team decided to test that possibility, by first testing GLP-1.

In one preclinical study, they let rats self-administer heroin or saline for 6 hours a day for 11 days, followed by 13 days of abstinence in their home cages. After this, the rats were injected with one dose of liraglutide at 0.3 milligrams per kilogram or with saline solution. Six hours later, they were placed back into the test chamber with no drug available and tested for heroin seeking. The team began by inducing seeking by exposing the rats to various drug-related cues. Next, after the rats' seeking slowed because they were not receiving any heroin, the rats were injected with a single IV infusion of heroin to trigger drug-induced seeking. Finally, the rats were injected with the stressor yohimbine to elicit stress-induced seeking.

In the case of seeking triggered by drug-related cues, Grigson's team found that the rats with a history of heroin self-administration and that were pretreated with saline did a lot of seeking in response to these cues, but the rats that had been treated with liraglutide demonstrated significantly reduced seeking behavior. Similarly, the infusion of heroin triggered the saline-treated rats to contact the empty spout in an attempt to get more, while the liraglutide-treated subjects did not exhibit this behavior. Finally, when the animals were injected with yohimbine, the saline-treated animals exhibited seeking behavior, while those treated with liraglutide did not (Douton et al., 2022). In short, the GLP-1R agonist blocked all three "roads to relapse"—those elicited by cues, the heroin itself, and stress.

Grigson's team saw similar results for fentanyl. Male rats that had self-administered fentanyl and then were abstinent could resist relapse if they had been treated with liraglutide (Urbanik et al., 2022), and this has been shown to be true in female rats as well (Urbanik et al., 2025). Another study showed that liraglutide administered chronically across the abstinence period instead of in a single acute dose just before the test still worked to reduce heroin seeking, particularly in rats that had a history of high drug taking (Evans et al., 2022). This is important for possible human application, as the drug regimen in this experiment more closely resembles the treatment that individuals with an opioid use disorder would undergo.

Grigson has also worked with a clinical team to examine GLP-1R agonists for the treatment of opioid use disorder in human participants in a phase 2 clinical trial.[1] These participants went through medically assisted withdrawal, and they had the choice of having medications for opioid use disorder (MOUD) with buprenorphine/naloxone or not. The patients were then randomized to receive either placebo or liraglutide once a day (with the dosage increasing across 18 days), then they were taken off the treatment for 2 days, and 30 days later they were followed up with a phone call.

During the course of the treatment, Grigson's team measured blood glucose, body weight, and ambient drug craving using ecological momentary assessment, a smartphone app that asks questions four times a day about cravings, nausea, mood, and sleep. The researchers also measured blood

---

[1] For more information on the phase 2 clinical trial, please see https://clinicaltrials.gov/study/NCT04199728?term=NCT04199728 (accessed December 30, 2024).

pressure, heart rate, respiratory rate, and blood oxygen saturation at the start of the study, with every increase in dose, and at the end of the study.

Grigson's team recruited 25 individuals who were randomized into treatment groups. Twenty of them were tested with the ecological momentary assessment. Thirteen chose to have the buprenorphine/naltrexone MOUD, of which six were given placebo and seven received the liraglutide; of the seven who did not choose MOUD, four received a placebo and three got liraglutide. The liraglutide proved to be safe. It did not adversely affect body weight, blood glucose, or cardiovascular function in the 3-week study.

To measure efficacy, Grigson's group collected 596 data points across 202 days. They used the Desire for Drug Scale, which asks responders to rate three aspects of desire for drugs on a five-point Likert scale—whether drugs intruded on their thoughts that day, whether they have missed the feeling that drugs can give them, and whether they have thought about how satisfying drugs can be (Love et al., 1998). The score on the scale is the average of the responses to the three items, which range from 0 for strongly disagree to 4 for strongly agree. The scale, originally developed for alcohol use disorder, has been shown to be a valid measure for opioid use disorder as well (Cleveland et al., 2021).

The team's analysis of the data showed that individuals who were treated with liraglutide reported 40 percent less opioid craving than those that were treated with placebo, Grigson said. Importantly, she added, they found that the GLP-1 agonist was significantly effective beginning with the lowest dose. The individuals on placebo experienced increased craving as the day wore on from morning through evening, while the craving remained relatively flat throughout the day for those in the liraglutide group, so that they reported having significantly less craving than the placebo group in the afternoon and evening. Both groups reported high levels of stress, but for the individuals on the placebo, their higher levels of stress were associated with higher levels of craving, which was not the case for those taking the liraglutide.

The clinical trial did have some limitations, Grigson said, such as its sample size, the fact that the population was mostly male and mostly White, and that it was done in a residential setting. However, it did clearly indicate that the GLP-1R agonist was effective in reducing opioid craving, beginning with the lowest dose. It was effective at times of high risk, specifically the afternoon and evening, it was effective with or without the MOUD, and it dissociated craving from stress.

Looking to the future, Grigson concluded, more research is needed to understand the optimal treatment, such as how to identify the ideal drug, dose, treatment regimen, drug combinations, treatment parameters, and concomitant treatments to address psychological and physiological issues.

USING REAL-WORLD EVIDENCE TO STUDY THE USE OF SEMAGLUTIDE IN TREATING SUBSTANCE USE DISORDERS

Carrying out randomized controlled trials (RCTs) to test the effectiveness of GLP-1R agonists in treating substance use disorders is very expensive and time-consuming, noted Rong Xu, a professor of biomedical informatics and founding director of the Center for Artificial Intelligence in Drug Discovery at Case Western Reserve University. She and her team have instead taken advantage of the large amounts of real-world data available in a large health care database to emulate RCTs and generate information about the effectiveness of these drugs much more quickly and less expensively than can be done with actual RCTs.

Xu's team uses longitudinal data from TriNetX, a Boston-based company with access to data on 250 million unique patients from 120 health organizations across 19 countries. Xu's studies have focused on U.S. data, which covers 117 million patients from 66 health care organizations across all 50 states. The data are very rich, including demographics, social determinants of health, genomic data, test diagnoses, and medication procedures, with up to 20 years of patient history. The health records are de-identified, so the patients are anonymous.

A randomized clinical trial generally has seven components, Xu said: eligibility criteria, treatment strategies, treatment assignment, outcomes, follow-ups, causal contrast of interest, and statistical analysis. In emulating such a trial with real-world data, she continued, the biggest challenge is the treatment assignment. "For randomized clinical trials, you randomly assign the treatment strategy to a participant," she said, but this isn't possible for real-world data. Instead, her team uses propensity score matching to make sure the exposure cohort and the comparison cohort are similar in terms of their characteristics. The resulting emulation trial generally costs less than $1 million to perform on potentially millions of patients, while a randomized trial with hundreds of patients will typically cost $10 million to $50 million, Xu said.

The first study her team published using this approach looked at the GLP-1R agonist semaglutide and its effects on alcohol use disorder (Wang et al., 2024a). In that study they looked at four cohorts that each had 5,000–80,000 participants: patients with obesity and no prior alcohol use disorder (AUD), patients with type 2 diabetes and no prior AUD, patients with obesity and preexisting AUD, and patients with type 2 diabetes and preexisting AUD. In the two obesity cohorts, they compared patients given semaglutide versus patients given other types of weight loss drugs, while in the two diabetes cohorts they compared patients given semaglutide versus patients given other anti-diabetes drugs. In the two cohorts whose members had no existing AUD, the outcome of interest was a first-time diagnosis of

AUD, while in the two cohorts whose members had preexisting AUD, the outcome of interest was a subsequent medical encounter for AUD. The patients were followed for 12 months, and the time at which an outcome of interest occurred, if it did, was recorded.

After analyzing the data, Xu's group found that semaglutide was associated with a decreased risk for developing AUD by 50 percent among those who had never had the disorder and a risk for recurrent AUD decreased by 56 percent among those who had previously been diagnosed with AUD. For type 2 diabetes, the corresponding decreases were 44 percent and 40 percent (Wang et al., 2024a). It is possible, Xu said, that the decreases were lower in the case of diabetes because semaglutide was generally prescribed at a higher dosage for obesity than for diabetes.

Xu's group used the same study approach—four cohorts covering both obesity and diabetes and both individuals with a preexisting cannabis use disorder (CUD) and those with no history of the disorder—to look at the effects of semaglutide on CUD (Wang et al., 2024b). The results were similar: Among patients with obesity there was a 44 percent reduction in the number of cases of incident CUD and a 38 percent reduction in recurrent CUD. Among those with type 2 diabetes there was a 60 percent reduction in incident CUD and a 34 percent reduction in recurrent CUD.

In a third study they examined the effect of semaglutide on tobacco use disorder (TUD). In this case, they looked at more than 200,000 patients with type 2 diabetes and preexisting TUD. They did not look at patients with obesity because the relationship between smoking and losing weight would introduce too many confounding factors. Patients on semaglutide were compared with patients on each of seven other anti-diabetes drugs, including first-generation GLP-1R agonists. They found that semaglutide was consistently associated with a reduction of 12–30 percent in diagnoses of TUD in all the stratified populations, a 40–70 percent reduction in the prescription of smoking cessation medication prescription, and a 20–30 percent reduction for smoking cessation counseling (Wang et al., 2024c).

In a fourth study they looked at patients with type 2 diabetes and a preexisting opioid use disorder and found that being treated with semaglutide was associated with about a 50 percent reduction in the risk of opioid overdose when compared with other anti-diabetes medications (Wang et al., 2024d). A fifth study found semaglutide to be associated with a 50–80 percent reduction in risk for suicidal ideation in both patients with obesity and patients with type 2 diabetes (Wang et al., 2024e).

In closing, Xu said that when her group used real-world data to emulate randomized clinical trials, they found evidence supporting potential benefits of using semaglutide for treating multiple substance use disorders. The limitations of the work include the fact that real-world data have various confounders and biases, and trial emulations do not necessarily capture the outcomes from randomized clinical trials. Thus, in the future it will be necessary to carry out RCTs to verify the findings of these trial emulations, she said. Future work should also be aimed at understanding the mechanisms of action involved in GLP-1R agonists' ameliorating substance use disorders.

DISCUSSION

Effects of GLP-1R Agonists on Endogenous GLP-1 Levels

Brian Fiske brought up the DPP-4 data that Farokhnia had discussed and said it reminded him of a question from an earlier session concerning whether it might not be feasible to elevate endogenous GLP-1. Could the system be so tightly regulated, he asked, that it would essentially be impossible to increase endogenous GLP-1 enough to meaningfully stimulate the GLP-1 system without directly targeting the receptors themselves? Is that what the DPP-4 data imply?

"That's what we are thinking right now," Farokhnia replied. Since the experiments he talked about were very preliminary, his group is carrying out more experiments, including measuring endogenous GLP-1 levels to see how much the levels are increased by the DPP-4 inhibitors. And even if a DPP-4 inhibitor did increase the levels of exogenous GLP-1 levels, he continued, it is quite possible that this increase would not help in controlling substance use disorders since although DPP-4 inhibitors regulate blood glucose levels in patients, they do not really affect appetite or eating.

In response to a question on the effects of GLP-1R agonists on the central norepinephrine system, Jerlhag said her lab has looked at that issue for various agonists, and the only one they have found so far that affects that system is liraglutide. "We found that it affected noradrenaline in prefrontal cortex, but not in any other areas," she said.

Then, on the issue of whether GLP-1R agonists paired with GIP analogs might have a greater effect together than either has by itself, Jerlhag said her lab has done extensive studies on that, and they have found a strong positive effect from the dual agonist tirzepatide. It appears tirzepatide has a somewhat stronger effect than semaglutide, though the stronger effect is mainly visible in females.

Possible Mechanisms in the Actions of GLP-1R Agonists for Substance Use Disorder

Serena Jingchuan Guo, an assistant professor in the Department of Pharmaceutical Outcomes and Policy at the University of Florida College of Pharmacy, asked about the existence of studies looking into the mechanisms behind the addiction prevention effects of GLP-1R agonists. As background, she described a targeted trial emulation study that her group had carried out with a national sample of Medicare beneficiaries. In the patients with a preexisting opioid use disorder, the researchers found that GLP-1R agonists had a modest protective effect against the opioid overdose, but in patients with no history of opioid use disorder or opioid overdose history, they found that, compared with DPP-4, the GLP-1R agonist was associated with an increased risk of newly diagnosed opioid use disorder. "We haven't submitted it for publication yet," she said, "because we couldn't find a mechanism study to support the biological possibility."

Xu said that in an unpublished study of semaglutide in patients with type 2 diabetes, when they used AI to identify the targets of semaglutide in substance use disorder, they found that semaglutide has a lot of off-target effects beyond GLP-1 receptors. Indeed, she said, the top effect was not with a GLP-1 receptor but instead was something related to a brain reward system.

Regarding the effects Guo saw, Grigson suggested that "one might wonder if the drug is experienced as less reinforcing for the new users, and they might have been compensating by trying a higher dose."

In response to a question about whether some of the effects of the GLP-1R agonists on substance use might be due to aversion in the same way that reduced food intake for some of these drugs is related to nausea in humans, Jerlhag said her team used very low doses in their studies, and tests showed that these doses did not appear to affect nausea at all. Furthermore, the various GLP-1R agonists are consistent in their reduction in the rewarding effects of alcohol, especially by dopamine release.

Schmidt expanded on that answer. "I don't think that the cocaine-exposed brain necessarily reacts the same way to these drugs that a drug-naive brain would," he said, which is supported by preclinical studies. In their cocaine studies, for example, they have identified both systemic and intracranial doses of GLP-1R agonists that selectively reduce cocaine seeking and don't affect food intake or produce malaise-like effects. "I think we're taking a very dopamine-centric view of the mechanisms here," he continued, "but there are certainly other circuits that are going to be involved." In particular, one nicotine study showed that activating GLP-1 receptors in the medial habenula–interpeduncular nucleus pathway increases the aversive effects of nicotine (Tuesta et al., 2017). So there are clearly other things than just dopamine involved in both the reward and aversion circuits in the brain, Schmidt said.

Grigson added that in an unpublished preclinical study she found that the GLP-1R agonist reduced evidence of naloxone-induced withdrawal (i.e., aversive faces to a taste cue that has been paired with naloxone-induced withdrawal). It is possible, she said, that the agonist's effects involve not just reducing the rewarding aspects of a drug but also the aversiveness of the craving for the drug. "We'll need more work to demonstrate that, though," she said.

Matthew Hayes asked about the role of stress in addiction and relapse, and Farokhnia said that there is a long line of literature showing that different types of stress and stress neuropeptides do trigger relapse and drug-seeking behavior. However, Farokhnia continued, "like the link with GLP-1, I don't think there has been a lot of work in the substance use arena. As everyone said, it's been very dopamine-centric so far."

A workshop participant asked whether substance use might affect the blood–brain barrier and alter the access of a GLP-1R agonist to the brain. Leggio noted that, similar to patients with Alzheimer's disease or Parkinson's disease, there is some evidence that the blood–brain barrier is disrupted in people with substance use disorder. Jerlhag added that in her tests on alcohol-drinking rats, fluorescently marked semaglutide was binding into the nucleus accumbens, which had not been shown in regular rats. That is an indication, she said, that semaglutide might pass more deeply into the brain, at least in rodents.

Other Possible Factors Involved in GLP-1R Efficacy

Alexandra Sinclair pointed to the studies that found the GLP-1R agonists to be effective against alcohol use disorder only in a subgroup that had obesity, and she also noted that epidemiological studies of the efficacy of GLP-1R agonists against substance use disorder tended to have data mainly from patients with obesity because they were the most likely to be prescribed one of the agonists. Given that, she said, what is known about possible differences in efficacy between individuals with and without obesity? To Farokhnia's understanding, the only clinical trial testing GLP-1R agonists on alcohol use disorder is the one he described in his presentation. That trial did find that people with a high BMI had a better response, but since it is the only such trial so far, it is too soon to know for sure whether that relationship between BMI and response will hold up. In their ongoing clinical trial, they are recruiting a wider range of participants, he said, but safety considerations keep them from recruiting people with a BMI below 25 because of concerns they might get too thin. Still, he concluded, "it's very plausible to think that people with higher BMI may respond better to these medications."

Leggio wrapped up the discussion session by responding to an online question from a workshop participant who asked about the social effects that GLP-1R agonists might have in humans. "Addiction is a complex disease where there are many social determinants," Leggio said. He added that one of the main challenges relative to these drugs, in addition to determining whether they work in people with addiction, will be implementing them at the community level. "Today we do have medications approved by the FDA to treat addiction, but they're only used for 2 percent to 20 percent of the patients," he said. "So, think about if this was a cancer workshop, and I was telling [you] today that we only treat 2 percent to 20 percent of people with cancer. That would be unacceptable." Given that, Leggio said, people in the field should also be thinking about implementation and the social implications for their patients.

6

Neurodegenerative Disorders and Other Emerging Areas

HIGHLIGHTS

- GLP-1R agonists have been evaluated across multiple preclinical neurodegenerative and neuropsychiatric disorder models and have been found highly promising. Clinical trials of GLP-1R agonists for the treatment of Parkinson's disease have had mixed results, but their results, combined with the results of preclinical research, indicate that the drugs have enough promise for research to continue. The agonists are also being tested in clinical trials of Alzheimer's disease. (Athauda, Greig, Hölscher)
- For GLP-1R agonists being considered for treatment of brain disorders and injuries, an important consideration is how well they cross the blood–brain barrier. (Athauda, Hölscher)
- Some recently developed dual agonists can cross the blood–brain better than previous GLP-1R agonists and, in animal studies, are better at protecting the brain than the older single agonists. (Hölscher)
- GLP-1R agonists show promise in treating the raised intracranial pressure associated with idiopathic intracranial hypertension and traumatic brain injury, headache and migraine pain, neuropathic pain, and the raised intraocular pressure that can lead to glaucoma. (Sinclair)

continued

- Biomarkers can play a valuable role in the development of GLP-1R agonists, particularly in serving as surrogate endpoints to evaluate their efficacy in treating various neurodegenerative disorders. (Jawidzik)

NOTE: This list is the rapporteurs' summary of points made by the individual speakers identified, and the statements have not been endorsed or verified by the National Academies of Sciences, Engineering, and Medicine. They are not intended to reflect a consensus among workshop participants.

The action of glucagon-like peptide-1 receptor (GLP-1R) drugs in treating neurodegenerative disorders and other disorders is currently receiving a great deal of attention, said Edwin George, a clinical reviewer in the Office of New Drugs in the Food and Drug Administration's (FDA) Center for Drug Evaluation and Research. He listed three objectives for the session focused on those uses: (1) to review the current state of knowledge regarding the mechanisms of action of GLP-1R agonists and their use in treating neurodegenerative disorders, pain syndromes, and other central nervous system (CNS) disorders; (2) to discuss the available scientific evidence on the clinical efficacy of GLP-1R agonists for treating various CNS disorders; and (3) to discuss the challenges relating to these issues, including knowledge gaps, clinical trial design, and biomarker development.

GLP-1 RECEPTOR ACTIVITY IN NEURODEGENERATIVE DISORDERS

Explaining why researchers studying neurodegenerative diseases are interested in GLP-1R agonists, Nigel Greig, who leads the Drug Design and Development Section within the Translational Gerontology Branch at the National Institute on Aging at the National Institutes of Health (NIH), said that there are many commonalities between type 2 diabetes and neurodegenerative disorders, particularly related to cell death mechanisms. And, indeed, a large study of patients being treated for type 2 diabetes found that those treated with a GLP-1R agonist were 60 percent less likely to develop Parkinson's disease than those given glitazones, a standard treatment for insulin resistance (Brauer et al., 2020). Thus, researchers have been examining the role of GLP-1 receptor activity in neurodegenerative disorders.

GLP-1 receptors are distributed throughout the brain, Greig said, including in the amygdala, hippocampus, and hypothalamus (Lu et al., 2014), and they are found on neurons, epithelial cells of the choroid plexus

(Botfield et al., 2017), and microglia and astrocytes (Jia et al., 2015). Two decades of research in cellular and animal models have found that GLP-1R agonists have neurotrophic, neuroprotective, and anti-inflammatory actions and mitigate brain insulin resistance. Thus, they have potential to treat a wide variety of neurological disorders and injuries.

The key question, Greig continued, is whether these actions of GLP-1R agonists seen in cellular and animal models translate to humans. Answering this question will require addressing other questions, such as which agonists should be evaluated and when in the disease process should they be evaluated. For an overview of the field, he recommended reading a recent publication by Kopp and colleagues (2024).

Quickly reviewing a number of studies, Greig said that research conducted in lab animals indicates that GLP-1 receptors are expressed across the lifespan and in disease states, such as a rodent model for Parkinson's disease. Corresponding studies in humans found that GLP-1 receptors were found in the substantia nigra in people with Parkinson's disease. In short, the receptors are expressed across age and disease state.

When cells with GLP-1 receptors are put in culture and exposed to GLP-1R agonists, the result is a stronger phenotypic expression, said Greig; so if, for example, the cell expresses tyrosine hydroxylase, administration of the agonist results in more tyrosine hydroxylase being expressed. The GLP-1R agonists also provide a protective effect, keeping cells alive when they are treated with chemicals that would otherwise kill them (Li et al., 2009).

Turning briefly to the pathways through which GLP-1R activation has its effects, Greig said that they are well known (see, e.g., Kopp et al., 2022). To find out which pathways are involved in neurotrophic and neuroprotective actions, one can put selective inhibitors of the various pathways into a cell culture and observe which ones prevent the effects of the GLP-1R activation. And once these pathways have been identified, their markers can be used in human studies as biomarkers of target engagement by assaying brain-derived exosomes from plasma (Athauda et al., 2019).

Switching to research done on GLP-1R agonists in preclinical models of Parkinson's disease, Greig first described work done on the MPTP (1-methyl-4-phenyl-1,2,3,6-tetrahydropyridine) mouse model of Parkinson's disease, which is created by exposing a mouse to the dopamine cell poison MPTP. When MPTP mice are treated with the GLP-1R agonist exendin-44, the drug protects the tyrosine hydroxylase–positive neurons in the mouse's brain and preserves the levels of dopamine and metabolites in those neurons (Li et al., 2009).

A second model is the MitoPark mouse, a progressive Parkinson's disease model created by deleting TFAM (transcription factor A, mitochondrial) in midbrain dopamine neurons. A careful study of the effects of a GLP-1R agonist in that mouse model found that the drug improved the mouse's motor abilities and increased motivated behavior, increased dopamine levels, and protected neurons. The authors of the study (Wang et al., 2021) concluded that early administration of this GLP-1R agonist (PT320, a sustained-release version of exenatide) could be an important neuroprotective therapeutic strategy against Parkinson's disease.

Summarizing, Greig said that GLP-1R agonists have been evaluated across multiple preclinical neurodegenerative and neuropsychiatric disorder models and, largely, have been found highly promising. Combining two or more agonists together, as in unimolecular multiagonists that target the receptors for GLP-1 and glucose-dependent insulinotropic polypeptide (GIP), is more effective than using a single GLP-1R agonist, although only if they are taken up by the brain. Furthermore, in human clinical trials of Parkinson's disease, GLP-1R agonists are demonstrating promise, and the agonists are also being tested in clinical trials of Alzheimer's disease. In the future, Greig said, it would be valuable to test GLP-1R agonists against other neurodegenerative diseases and brain injury with a focus on finding the best agents and best times in the disease process to initiate treatment.

GLP-1R AGONISTS IN TREATING PARKINSON'S DISEASE

Building on Greig's discussion of preclinical data on GLP-1R agonists and Parkinson's disease, Dilan Athauda, a consultant neurologist and neuroscientist at University College London, spoke about the clinical data concerning the efficacy of using the agonists in treating Parkinson's disease. He began by noting, as Greig had, that cohort studies have found that patients taking GLP-1R agonists for type 2 diabetes have a significantly reduced risk of developing Parkinson's disease (Brauer et al., 2020; Svenningsson et al., 2016; Tang et al., 2024).

In light of those findings, a clinical pilot study was carried out on 44 patients with Parkinson's disease. The patients were an average of 60 years old, had had Parkinson's for an average of 10 years, and were on an average of 980 mg of the dopamine precursor levodopa daily. In the study they were given either the GLP-1R agonist exenatide or a control treatment for 12 months. They were tested at baseline, 6 months, 12 months, and 14 months on a variety of motor and cognitive tests, and the group given the exenatide scored significantly better on both types of tests than the control group. The drug was well tolerated, and when the patients were retested at 96 weeks, or about 22 months, the improvement in the treatment group versus the controls had been maintained (Aviles-Olmos et al., 2013).

Athauda and his group followed that up with their own study examining the effects of a different form of exenatide on Parkinson's disease. Their 60 patients had experienced somewhat less advanced Parkinson's, on average, but saw a similar effect on motor control, with the treatment group seeing improved motor control and the placebo group continuing to get worse over the course of the study (see Figure 6-1). In this case, however, there were no significant differences in cognitive measures (Athauda et al., 2017). Looking more closely, the researchers found reduced dopamine terminal loss in the brains of the patients, improved neuropsychiatric symptoms such as mood and emotional well-being, and evidence that the drug (when injected) crossed the blood–brain barrier and enhanced insulin signaling in the brain (Athauda et al., 2018, 2019).

Other studies have not had such positive results. A 2022 study by the biotech company Peptron Inc. examined the effects of a sustained-release form of exenatide, PT320, over 48 weeks and found no significant effect on motor control, although there was at least one significant improvement in a quality-of-life measure. The results have not been published, Athauda said, though they were described in a press release (Chang, 2022). The company said it believes there was enough of a signal to continue its studies.

A small study of liraglutide, another GLP-1R agonist, found no significant improvement in motor control, although it did see improvement in some nonmotor measures as well as in some quality-of-life scores (Malatt et al., 2022). A study of the effects of NLY01, a PEGylated[1] form of exenatide, on a group of 225 people who had Parkinson's disease for an average of only 1 year found that 36 weeks of treatment had no effect on motor function or nonmotor measures (McGarry et al., 2024). Another

---

[1] PEGylation is the act of attaching polyethylene glycol (PEG) chains to a molecule. It is often used with drugs to increase the amount of time they remain in the bloodstream.

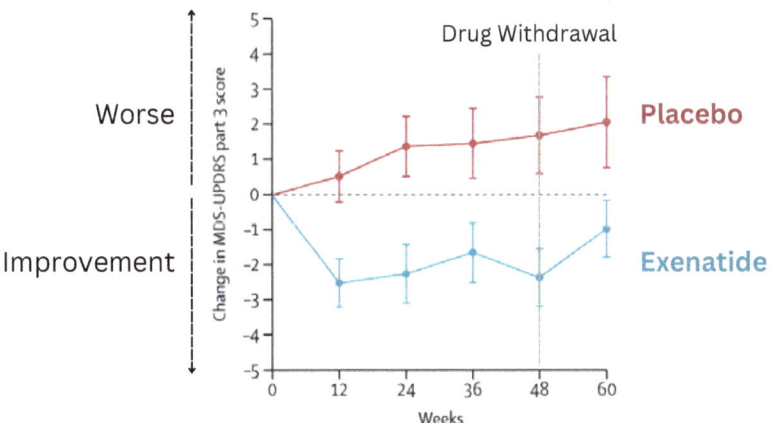

FIGURE 6-1 Effect of exenatide on Parkinson's disease.
NOTE: MDS-UPSDRS part 3 = Movement Disorder Society Unified Parkinson's Disease Rating Scale (MDS-UPDRS) part III.
SOURCE: Presented by Dilan Athauda on September 10, 2024. Adapted from Athauda et al., 2017. Reprinted from *The Lancet*, with permission from Elsevier.

trial of a GLP-1R agonist, lixisenatide, for treatment of early Parkinson's disease did find an effect on motor function, with the treatment group maintaining their score and the placebo group getting worse, although there were no significant changes on secondary outcomes (Meissner et al., 2024).

Given the varying results of these trials, Athauda asked, should researchers continue to explore this class of drugs for use to treat Parkinson's disease? In light of the strong preclinical evidence, he said, he believes that GLP-1R agonists should have an effect on Parkinson's disease, and the fact that the clinical trials have used different methods and different drugs and doses justifies additional research. A major question is which of these drugs cross the blood–brain barrier; while exenatide, for instance, does seem to cross the barrier and get into cerebrospinal fluid (Athauda et al., 2017) liraglutide does not (Christensen et al., 2015).

Looking forward, Athauda recommended collaboration and data sharing across GLP-1 clinical trials to identify gaps in knowledge and biomarkers of target engagement. He also said that the newer double and triple agonists (such as GLP-1 combined with GIP and glucagon) show greater promise and may prove to be more effective against Parkinson's disease.

PENETRATION OF THE BLOOD–BRAIN BARRIER BY GLP-1 CLASS DRUGS AND NEUROPROTECTION

Christian Hölscher discussed the importance of GLP-1 class drugs being able to pass through the blood–brain barrier if they are to help treat neurodegenerative diseases.

He began by describing the potential value of these drugs. GLP-1 is a growth factor that normalizes energy use in the brain, reduces chronic inflammation, and greatly enhances neuronal survival and synaptic activity. Preclinical studies have shown GLP-1R agonists to have good effects on both Parkinson's disease and Alzheimer's disease; for instance, more than a decade ago the diabetes drug liraglutide had positive effects in a mouse model of Alzheimer's disease (McClean et al., 2011). And a 12-month, double-blind, placebo-controlled phase 2 clinical study that Hölscher was involved with found improved cognition and reduced brain shrinkage in Alzheimer's patients treated with liraglutide (Femminella et al., 2019). It offered a proof of concept that GLP-1 analogs are effective in the clinic, Hölscher said, but the effect was limited, and better drugs are needed. And indeed, he added, two phase 3 trials are now examining the effects of semaglutide in Alzheimer's patients, so more information should be available soon.

To illustrate the importance of drugs being able to get past the blood–brain barrier, Hölscher referred to two of the same trials that Athauda had discussed. Athauda and colleagues (2017) had found that a once-weekly form of exendin-4 given over 7 months significantly improved motor function in patients with Parkinson's disease, while McGarry and colleagues (2024) reported that NYL01, a PEGylated form of exendin-4, given over 36 weeks had no effect on Parkinson's patients. The difference could be due to NYL01, which is created by adding polyethylene glycol (PEG) polymer chains to the exendin-4 molecule, being too large to cross the blood–brain barrier, Hölscher explained. An experiment by Yun and colleagues (2018) demonstrated this explicitly.

This is a problem for the current generation of GLP-1R agonists, Hölscher said, given that they are designed to treat type 2 diabetes and to stay in the bloodstream as long as possible so that they do not enter the brain well. For that reason, his group has designed some new peptide drugs that are designed to cross the blood–brain barrier more quickly; they are dual agonists, activating both the GLP-1 receptor and the glucose-dependent insulinotropic polypeptide receptor. GIP is a peptide hormone that acts a growth factor, much like GLP-1, and GIP analogs have been shown to have neuroprotective effects in both Alzheimer's and Parkinson's patients.

Recent work has shown that the dual agonists developed by his group enter the brain effectively and, in many cases, more quickly than the traditional GLP-1R agonists such as exenatide and lixisenatide (Rhea et al., 2023; Salameh et al., 2020). (Both liraglutide and semaglutide are particularly poor at crossing the blood–brain barrier and did not enter the brain in significant level in these studies.) Tests in the MPTP mouse model of Parkinson's disease showed that two of the dual agonists developed by Hölscher's group, DA-JC4 and DA-CH5, were neuroprotective (Feng et al., 2018).

In conclusion, Hölscher said, the fact that these dual agonists can cross the blood–brain better than previous GLP-1R agonists and are better at protecting the brain than single agonists, as demonstrated by animal studies, supports the idea that the new dual agonists "will be much more effective in the clinic." The group's most promising dual agonist, DA-CH5, has now entered phase 1 clinical trials.

TREATING IDIOPATHIC INTRACRANIAL HYPERTENSION AND OTHER PRESSURE-RELATED DISORDERS

Alexandra Sinclair discussed the potential of GLP-1R agonists in treating disorders related to increased pressure in the brain and the eyes. In addition to their better-known anti-obesity and neuroprotective effects, GLP-1R agonists also reduce intracranial pressure, interocular pressure, and pain from migraines and neuropathy. This makes it possible that these agonists could be used in the treatment of such things as idiopathic intracranial hypertension, traumatic brain injury (TBI), space-flight-associated neuro-ocular syndrome, and glaucoma, as well as migraines and neuropathy. Furthermore, she added, the fact that these agonists can act against multiple issues at once broadens their potential clinical utility (see Figure 6-2).

Preclinical research in her lab has determined where GLP-1R agonists are expressed in the brain, traced the neurological pathways by which they work, and shown that one such agonist, exenatide, does a better job of reducing intracranial pressure in lab animals than other known drugs (Botfield et al., 2017). Importantly, she added, the way GLP-1R agonists reduce intracranial pressure is independent of what has caused the pressure, meaning that the agonists can be effective for any condition alleviated by reducing intracranial pressure, including idiopathic intracranial hypertension, TBI, and stroke with raised intracranial pressure.

Focusing on idiopathic intracranial hypertension, she said it is a disease that affects almost exclusively women between puberty and menopause who have obesity. The disease is thought to be driven by metabolic syndrome and excess androgens. People with it have increased intracranial pressure, and the resulting pressure on the optical nerve can lead to blindness as well as headaches. It is a rare disease, occurring in about 2 per 100,000 people, and so far, there are no effective drugs to treat it. In a phase 2 clinical trial, Sinclair's group found that exenatide produced a significant reduction in intercranial pressure in adults with idiopathic intracranial hypertension; the pressure reduction was independent of weight loss, and the treatment also significantly reduced the frequency of headaches in the subjects (Krajnc et al., 2023: Mitchell et al., 2023).

Turning to the treatment of migraine and headache pain, Sinclair said that GLP-1R expression has been found in the trigeminocervical complex, which is known to play a key role in migraines, and that in a migraine mouse model, a GLP-1R agonist reduced pain by stimulating interleukin 10 (Halloum et al., 2024; Jing et al., 2021, 2023). A small human trial, whose results have not been published, found that a GLP-1R agonist

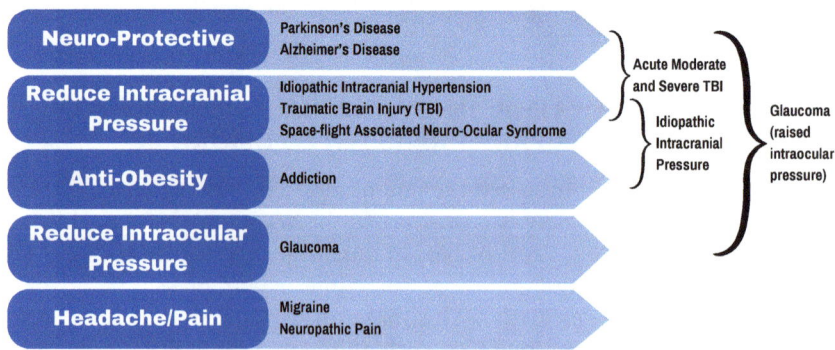

FIGURE 6-2 Effects of GLP-1R agonists on the central nervous system.
NOTE: GLP-1R = glucagon-like peptide-1 receptor; TBI = traumatic brain injury.
SOURCE: Presented by Alexandra Sinclair on September 10, 2024.

reduced headache frequency but not body mass index (BMI) in a group of 26 migraine patients with obesity.

On the topic of treating neuropathic pain with GLP-1R agonists, Sinclair said that there has been no clinical research, but some preclinical research indicates the agonists could be effective. A typical way that patients develop neuropathic pain is through diabetic or metabolic causes or injury leading to inflammation, and preclinical data indicate that GLP-1R agonists activate the GLP-1 receptors on microglia in the spinal dorsal horn, increasing interleukin 10 levels and reducing markers of inflammation. In mice models, a GLP-1R agonist reduced neuropathic pain and pain signaling.

Concerning TBI, Sinclair continued, the primary way it manifests its effects is through raised intracranial pressure, with leads to an inflammatory cascade and secondary injury, causing brain cell death and other poor outcomes. Preclinical data have shown that GLP-1R agonists have neuroprotective effects against moderate TBI. They attenuate inflammation and improve functional outcomes, including cognitive function (Zhang et al., 2020). However, no clinical trials have examined the use of GLP-1R agonists in treating TBI, nor have any studies examined epidemiological data.

By contrast, there is evidence in humans—from retrospective case reviews—that GLP-1R agonists can reduce intraocular pressure and lower the risk of glaucoma (Hallaj et al., 2025; Niazi et al., 2024; Sterling et al., 2023). This fits with preclinical data, which have found that GLP-1R agonists act in the retinal ganglion cells of the optic nerve to reduce inflammation, oxidative stress, and neuron death (Lawrence et al., 2023; Sterling et al., 2020).

In summary, Sinclair said, GLP-1R agonists may someday be used to treat more than just type 2 diabetes and obesity. They show promise in treating the raised intracranial pressure associated with idiopathic intracranial hypertension and TBI, headache and migraine pain, neuropathic pain, and the raised intraocular pressure that can lead to glaucoma. These wider uses, in turn, may create opportunities for more personalized medicine, as many patients present with more than one of these conditions, such as patients with obesity, diabetes, and migraines or glaucoma. The goal will be to tailor the drugs' effects to target specific patient subgroups depending on their comorbidities. This will require clever clinical trial designs and trials that are suitably powered.

BIOMARKERS IN DRUG DEVELOPMENT

Laura Jawidzik, the deputy director of the Division of Neurology 1 at the FDA's Center for Drug Evaluation and Research, provided an overview of the use of biomarkers in drug development. She began by stating that a biomarker is "a defined characteristic that is measured as an indicator of normal biological processes, pathogenic processes, or responses to an exposure or intervention, including therapeutic interventions." The types of biomarkers include molecular (such as a genetic test), histologic (such as a pathological assessment), radiographic (such as magnetic resonance image), or physiologic (such as blood pressure or an electroencephalogram). Biomarkers generally measure disease presence or status or aspects of response to treatment. However, a biomarker is not a measure of how a patient feels, functions, or survives (FDA-NIH Biomarker Working Group, n.d.).

The purposes for which biomarkers are used include making diagnoses, monitoring conditions, monitoring responses, predicting future states, making prognoses, assessing safety, and assessing susceptibility or risk, Jawidzik said. Then she offered a number of examples of biomarkers, including the SMN1 gene, which is used to diagnose spinal muscular atrophy; magnetic resonance imaging, which is used to monitor the status of multiple sclerosis; the ApoE4 gene, which serves as a marker for susceptibility to Alzheimer's disease; and the safety biomarker alanine transaminase, high levels of which indicate issues with the liver.

FDA urges drug developers to use biomarkers at all stages of drug development, Jawidzik said, from discovery through preclinical work and clinical trials and, finally, post marketing. Specifically, biomarkers can be used in proof-of-concept studies, such as to show that a drug is performing as expected; in selecting subjects for a trial, such as those who are more likely to respond to the treatment; in monitoring, as in looking for patients who may have adverse responses in the trial; and determining efficacy by, for instance, providing a surrogate endpoint for the primary outcome of interest. A surrogate endpoint, she explained, is an endpoint used in clinical trials as a substitute for a direct measure of how a patient feels, functions, or survives. There are two types: a validated surrogate endpoint, which has enough evidence supporting its predictive value that the FDA can use it directly in its approval decision; and a reasonably likely surrogate endpoint, which is supported by a mechanistic rationale or epidemiological data but not by enough clinical evidence to validate it, so it can be used only for accelerated approval of drugs or expedited access to medical devices. An example of a validated endpoint is blood pressure, as there is clear clinical evidence that lowering blood pressure will have health benefits, such as reducing the risk of stroke, so a drug can be approved merely on the basis of its ability to lower blood pressure.

Currently there are no validated surrogate endpoints for use as primary endpoints in clinical trials for drugs with neurological actions to treat neurological diseases, she said, but there are several reasonably likely surrogate endpoints. For example, a reduction in amyloid beta plaque was used for accelerated approval of lecanemab for Alzheimer's disease, and neurofilament light chain was used as a reasonably likely surrogate for the accelerated approval of tofersen for treatment of ALS (amyotrophic lateral sclerosis) in patients with the SOD1 mutation. In cases where a reasonably likely surrogate endpoint has been used for accelerated approval, the FDA still requires additional clinical data to show that there is a clinically meaningful outcome.

Biomarkers do not need to be qualified to be used in a drug development program, Jawidzik said, and the type and level of evidence needed to support a biomarker's use depends on the specific context. The FDA does have a Biomarker Qualification Program,[2] but it is generally used to prequalify biomarkers for use in drug development programs so that they can be used without further later qualification.

The FDA requires good scientific evidence for a biomarker to be used in drug development, and that evidence can take several forms. There should be a biological rationale for the use of the biomarker, if it is known. Assays should be analytically validated, and there should be a good understanding of potential sources of variability in the measurements. The relationship among the biomarker, outcome of interest, and treatment (where applicable) should be characterized for the particular proposed use. The types of data used to assess the strength of the association between the biomarker and its proposed outcome can include retrospective or prospective studies, registry data, and randomized controlled trial data.

In summary, Jawidzik said, the FDA encourages the use of biomarkers throughout the drug development life cycle, and it believes that biomarkers can help lead to the identification of more safe and effective therapies. George agreed, saying that a large focus in neurodegenerative diseases is early intervention and preventing neuronal death which reveals a need for biomarkers that can provide information on inflammation and changes in neuroprotective proteins.

DISCUSSION

In response to a question from George, Greig said that insulin resistance in the brain is linked with both Alzheimer's disease and Parkinson's disease, but the roles insulin resistance plays in these diseases are not clear. GLP-1R agonists trigger a whole series of cascades that relate to insulin resistance, neurotrophic actions, neuroprotective actions, anti-inflammatory actions, and many other actions, leading to an extremely complex system.

Matthew Coghlan, vice president and head of incretin portfolio science at Eli Lilly and Company, asked about the relative value of GIP analogs

---

[2] For more information about the FDA's Biomarker Qualification Program, see https://www.fda.gov/drugs/drug-development-tool-ddt-qualification-programs/biomarker-qualification-program (accessed November 9, 2024).

versus GLP-1R agonists. Hölscher responded that GIP analogs alone do have protective effects, but the effects are much greater when GIP is used in conjunction with GLP-1R agonists. Greig added that GIP can be very effective by itself with the right treatment regimen.

Mahin Khatami, retired from the National Cancer Institute, asked if long-term use of GLP-1R agonists might affect immune-responsive tissue, leading to cancer. Athauda answered that these drugs have been used for a couple of decades in humans, and epidemiological data show no evidence of an increased risk for various cancers, such as pancreatic cancer, thyroid cancer, or renal cancer. Sinclair agreed that long-term data have shown no indication of an increased cancer risk associated with these drugs.

Linda Rinaman asked how GLP-1R agonists exert their protective effect of sparing dopamine neurons from cell death given that these neurons do not have GLP-1 receptors. Greig responded that these neurons do have GLP-1 receptors, as has been shown in multiple ways. Hölscher said that the question of whether the dopaminergic neurons have GLP-1 receptors may not be particularly important anyway because these neurons are part of an entire system, with other types of cells that do have GLP-1 receptors. So if a GLP-1R agonist triggers anti-inflammatory responses in the surrounding cells, the dopaminergic cells would benefit from the agonist even if they themselves did not have the receptors. Rinaman responded that it does matter in the sense that it is important to understand the precise mechanisms by which the GLP-1R agonists exert their effects. Matt Hayes agreed that it is important to understand the mechanisms and said that there is good evidence that there are no GLP-1 receptors on dopamine neurons, at least in the ventral tegmental area.

Next, Hayes commented that as researchers design GLP-1 drugs that can cross the blood–brain barrier, they must take into account adverse effects that would accompany enhanced blood–brain barrier penetrance. So, he asked, what considerations should go into the design of these drugs in terms of this penetrance? Hölscher answered that it will depend on the desired purpose of the drug. Drugs to treat diabetes, for instance, should stay in the blood as long as possible and not cross the blood–brain barrier, whereas drugs for treating diseases of the central nervous system must be able to get into the brain. As for balancing the positive effects with adverse effects, he said that there are relatively few adverse effects to worry about; the drugs have proved to be safe and well tolerated, with minimal side effects. Hayes replied that nausea and vomiting are two well-known side effects of some GLP-1R agonists and that they should not be thought of as "minimal" because they are a leading reason why people stop taking prescribed drugs.

In summary, preclinical work indicates that GLP-1R agonists have potential for treating a number of neurodegenerative and neuropsychiatric disorders. Clinical research on the use of these agonists for Parkinson's disease has shown mixed results, while there have been promising results for the treatment of raised intracranial pressure, and clinical testing is ongoing for Alzheimer's disease. According to several participants, a key factor in the effectiveness of GLP-1R agonists may be how well they cross the blood–brain barrier.

7

Real-World Evidence, Accessibility, and Health Equity

HIGHLIGHTS

- Real-world data have great potential for addressing various questions concerning the use of glucagon-like peptide-1 receptor (GLP-1R) agonists in the treatment of various disorders. However, the use of real-world data in research also has a number of challenges. (Bian, Guo)
- One valuable way to use real-world data to gain insights into the effectiveness of GLP-1R agonists in treating various disorders is through trial emulation. Such data may also prove valuable in designing trial eligibility criteria. (Bian)
- The Food and Drug Administration is working to address current and future shortages in the supply of GLP-1R agonists. (Kosko)
- A variety of barriers make it more difficult for minorities and under-resourced populations to gain access to GLP-1R agonists to treat obesity, leading to barriers to inclusive and high-quality health care. (Stanford)

NOTE: This list is the rapporteurs' summary of points made by the individual speakers identified, and the statements have not been endorsed or verified by the National Academies of Sciences, Engineering, and Medicine. They are not intended to reflect a consensus among workshop participants.

Serena Jingchuan Guo began by providing the Food and Drug Administration (FDA) definitions of "real-world data" and "real-world evidence." Real-world data, she said, are data relating to patient health status or delivery of health care that are routinely collected from a variety of sources. Real-world evidence is clinical evidence derived from real-world data about the use and potential benefits or risks of a medical product. Such evidence might concern the effectiveness and safety of a drug or treatment, for example, or provide details about heterogeneity in treatment effect.

However, she continued, real-world clinical data are not collected for the purpose of providing evidence about the effectiveness of drugs or treatments, and there are many structural and methodological challenges with transforming such data into real-world clinical evidence. The challenges include missing clinical data, the often-poor organization of such data, and the fact that such data often do not provide the details researchers need to generate clinical evidence.

Despite those limitations, Guo continued, real-world evidence is uniquely positioned to address a number of important questions concerning the use of glucagon-like peptide-1 receptor (GLP-1R) agonists in the treatment of various disorders. These questions include the long-term effects of GLP-1R agonists on central nervous system (CNS) disorders, the safety profile of GLP-1R agonists in special populations (e.g., pregnant women, children, and aging populations), individualized treatment effects and precision dosing of GLP-1R agonists (e.g., for users with clinically high or low benefit or the balance of intended effect versus off-target effect), and head-to-head comparisons of the benefit-risk profile for different drugs (e.g., semaglutide versus tirzepatide).

Finally, Guo said, recent research has shown significant geographic and racial disparities in the use of GLP-1R agonists. For example, one study of the use of various glucose-lowering drugs, including GLP-1R agonist class drugs, for use in the treatment of type 2 diabetes found that non-Hispanic Black patients who were newly diagnosed with type 2 diabetes were only two-thirds as likely as newly diagnosed White patients to begin these drugs, even when clinical details were accounted for (Chen et al., 2024). The same study also found large geographic variation in how likely newly diagnosed patients were to use these drugs in the treatment of their diabetes.

Guo concluded her introduction by saying that the session would focus on three somewhat interrelated topics: real-world evidence, accessibility, and health equity.

USING REAL-WORLD DATA FOR TRIAL EMULATION

Jiang Bian, a professor of biomedical informatics at the University of Florida (UF) College of Medicine and the chief data scientist at UF Health, spoke about ways to use real-world data to carry out what he called "synthetic trials," which were very similar to the simulated trials that Rong Xu had discussed in the session on substance use disorders. Bian carries out his synthetic trials using a technique called trial emulation, which he described as a framework for dealing with the biases in observational data and achieving the sort of rigor one looks for in real trials.

As background, he noted that there is nothing new about using real-world data to draw conclusions about drug efficacy and safety (Concato and Corrigan-Curay, 2022; Sherman et al., 2016). For instance, the FDA has been doing postmarket surveillance with patients' electronic health records for years. "We need to figure out new ways to use this," he said. Other sorts of real-world data include health care claims data, tumor registry data, linked mother–baby data (i.e., birth records), and many others, and the various types of data are most powerful when they are linked to paint a more complete picture of patients. Importantly, Bian continued, there is an existing data infrastructure, both nationally and internationally, for dealing with real-world patient data. For example, PCORnet, which was founded by the Patient-Centered Outcomes Research Institute (PCORI), has data on about 100 million patients held in eight clinical data research networks. Trial emulation is one way to take advantage of those data, he added.

As an example of what is possible, Bian pointed to a study carried out by his team that looked at data from two large real-world datasets for more than 170 million patients over 10 years. The purpose of the study was to identify FDA-approved drugs that might be useful in treating Alzheimer's disease. Using machine learning, the researchers emulated trials for thousands of medications and found five medications who use was associated with a decreased use of developing Alzheimer's disease among patients with mild cognitive impairment (Zang et al., 2023).

In emulating a target trial, Bian said, one needs to specify seven key components of the target trial: the eligibility criteria, the treatment strategies being compared (including their start and end times), assignment procedures, the follow-up period, the outcome of interest, the causal contrasts of interest, and an analysis plan. Two components that are particularly important, he said, are the eligibility criteria and how outcomes in real-world data are defined.

To illustrate another way trial emulations can be used, Bian described a target trial emulation study that looked at how GLP-1R agonists might be used to treat Alzheimer's disease and related dementias. Using electronic health records from the OneFlorida+ dataset, they looked at a total of 33,858 patients with type 2 diabetes who were given various glucose-lowering drugs. Those who had received GLP-1R agonists had a reduced risk of developing Alzheimer's disease and related dementias, he said, but he emphasized that the trial emulation also made it possible to examine the drug's heterogeneous treatment effects across different subpopulations. For instance, if a patient had cardiovascular disease and some type of cerebrovascular disease, the treatment effect of the GLP-1R agonist was much bigger. "It does point [to] a way where you maybe design the drug for [a] specific subpopulation and where the real-world data can help you find that subpopulation," he said.

Bian then briefly described current work he is carrying out with Fei Wang of Weill Cornell Medicine on the use of real-world data in the design of trial eligibility criteria. The research, funded by the National Institute on Aging, is motivated by the issue of trial generalizability. Since trials are conducted in a constrained environment and do not match the target population in the real world, the goal of designing trial eligibility criteria is to minimize the gap between the trial subjects and the real-world target population to maximize the trial's generalizability as well as predicting potential outcomes and safety signals. Bian and Wang are working to apply explainable artificial intelligence methods to real-world data in order to assess the quantitative impacts of various eligibility criteria on clinical outcomes. One specific goal is to develop a prototype toolbox for eligibility design criteria.

Bian concluded by discussing some of the challenges in using real-world data. Misclassification issues are a major problem, for instance, as many clinicians are not accurate in coding diagnoses. One approach to solving this would be to develop more accurate computable phenotypes using informatics, though this would not completely prevent misclassification errors. Another major issue is that much of the information in electronic health records does not exist as structured data; some 80 percent of clinical information is in the form of free-text narratives, Bian said. Natural language processing may offer a solution to this problem. And there is a long list of other data types that are not readily accessible to researchers, such as imaging, genomics, and microbiome data. Ultimately, making these sorts of data easily available for research purposes will require a better data infrastructure, he said.

SHORTAGES OF GLP-1R AGONISTS

Robert Kosko, senior program management officer for the drug shortage staff at FDA and a commissioned officer in the U.S. Public Health Service, described FDA's role in ensuring the supply of drugs in the United States and, specifically, what is being done to deal with current shortages of GLP-1 class drugs.

He began by describing the FDA's role in ensuring the availability of safe and effective drugs in the United States. FDA staff works with manufacturers on both short-term and long-term strategies to address actual or potential supply interruptions, he said. "We don't want to just address the immediate issue, but we also want to ensure there are not continued issues that could impact future supply." The staff also works to develop a risk-benefit analysis for each drug shortage situation as well as to distribute information related to drug shortages by posting public information on the FDA website and reaching out to professional organizations and patient advocacy groups.

The staff has various tools to deal with a drug shortage situation, Kosko said. For instance, if a manufacturer notifies the FDA of a potential or actual shortage of concern, FDA staff can reach out to other manufacturers of the product to see if they can ramp up their own production. They can use regulatory flexibility to release a product to the market that does not meet the current FDA-approved specifications but with added safety controls or additional testing. They can also expedite the review of proposals and regulatory submissions. "And as a last resort," he said, "we will explore the potential importation of product to assist with a shortage situation. This requires careful evaluation of the product attributes, manufacturing facilities, and labeling."

Then Kosko turned to the current GLP-1R agonist supply situation in the United States, as of September 2024, when the workshop took place. The first GLP-1R agonist product shortage was posted on the FDA website at the end of March 2022, he said, and additional GLP-1R agonist products were added to the shortage website in August 2022, December 2022, July 2023, and April 2024. To date only the injectable formulations and not the oral formulations have experienced shortages in the United States, he said, and it appears that supply is now improving, with four of the injectable GLP-1R agonist products currently available in all of their approved forms, while most versions of the remaining products have limited availability.

He closed by talking about what the FDA is doing to assist with the supply of GLP-1R agonists. "First, we communicate on a regular basis with the sponsors regarding their current supply and demand, as well as projected demand and potential ways to increase supply," he said. "We also update availability information on our drug shortage website at least every 2 weeks and more frequently if additional supply information is provided by a sponsor." The staff responds to inquiries from patients and health care providers regarding these products with the most up-to-date availability information. Concerning the FDA's efforts to increase the supply of GLP-1R agonists, he said that the agency's main tactic is to expedite the review of proposals and regulatory submissions. "We have worked and continue to work with all sponsors of these products to provide feedback on any proposals as well as expedite the review of drug application supplements that can assist with increased supply." Finally, he said, FDA staff members participate in various working groups, attend workshops, and meet with their international regulatory counterparts to discuss current supply situations in their jurisdictions as well as best practices to address these shortages.

POTENTIAL BARRIERS AND SOLUTIONS TO WIDENING ACCESS TO GLP-1R AGONISTS FOR THE TREATMENT OF OBESITY

Fatima Cody Stanford discussed barriers to accessing GLP-1R agonists for the treating obesity and what might be done to overcome those barriers. Racial and ethnic minorities are the groups most likely to be affected by those barriers, she said, which is particularly important because those minorities are also often more affected by obesity. For instance, obesity affects more than 60 percent of Black women. And many minority patients with obesity find it difficult or impossible to gain access to GLP-1R agonists such as semaglutide or tirzepatide to treat their obesity. "I happen to work at one of the best-resourced hospitals in the world," she said, "and I can't get these to patients today." The situation is even worse for Medicaid and dual-eligible patients, that is, those who are eligible for both Medicare and Medicaid.

Stanford said the barriers to and solutions for widening access to GLP-1R agonists to treat obesity vary according to the actors involved. And, following an article she and colleagues recently published in *Nature Medicine*, she identified five groups of actors to consider: health care professionals, patients, insurance companies, governmental regulatory agencies, and drug manufacturers (Waldrop et al., 2024).

For health care professionals, she said, a major barrier is that a large percentage of them are not educated about obesity and perceive obesity as a consequence of personal choices, rather than as a disease. Stanford said potential solutions would include improved training within medical schools and residencies, cultural competency training, and training in implicit bias, weight bias, and the effects of weight stigmatization.

Patient-related barriers include the high cost of the medications, the need for long-term use, and safety concerns. The solutions Stanford suggested included helping patients to understand obesity as a disease requiring long-term therapy, improving how health care providers educate patients on the risks and benefits of starting and maintaining anti-obesity medications, and using better insurance coverage and third-party payer discounts to improve patients' access to these medications, regardless of their ability to pay.

Moving on to barriers related to insurance companies, Stanford pointed to the high cost of the medications and the need for long-term use. Potential solutions include facilitating greater access to the medications to improve cost sharing and removing drug therapies for obesity that have less efficacy and undesirable side effects, such as orlistat.

Barriers facing government regulatory agencies include both safety concerns and addressing stigma and bias related to obesity. According to Stanford, solutions include having these agencies follow medical society and drug manufacturer guidelines and evaluating more clinical data on safety and efficacy endpoints to support long-term use.

Finally, the barriers that drug manufacturers face include safety concerns and the fact that these treatments require long-term use, Stanford said. She emphasized the need for more studies specifically analyzing long-term use to provide clinical data on long-term safety and efficacy endpoints.

DISCUSSION

Challenges for Data Collection

Ellen Mowry asked how to overcome the confounding that will inevitably arise in any clinical study of GLP-1R agonists because people with higher socioeconomic status—who have access to better health care overall—will be far more likely than people with less money to have used these drugs. This could skew the results of any research on the benefits and risks of the drugs. Stanford replied that a group at Massachusetts General Hospital is planning to develop a data repository using data from individuals—typically with higher socioeconomic status—who are taking GLP-1R agonists. The group plans to start accumulating data from the point that individuals begin treatment with these drugs and working with collaborators in neurology, rheumatology, and other areas, record the results, analyze those results, and publish them. "I think this is going to be important for us to do across the board," she said. However, the data repository is likely to suffer from the same problem Mowry identified since most patients of lesser means will not be able to afford the drugs.

Bian commented that as long as some patients of limited means are receiving the drugs, researchers can use real-world data and data science methods to correct the bias. Also, he added, researchers might get funding to recruit specific minority cohorts to take these drugs to counteract some of the bias in the cohort.

Brian Fiske noted that GLP-1R agonists are starting to be prescribed for things other than type 2 diabetes and obesity, so data will start being accumulated in other places, such as by doctors treating CNS disorders. How can data be brought together from all these different specialists? Bian said that the problem is not so much collecting data, since the data can be found in electronic health records and prescription-dispensing records, and nationally a great deal of effort is going into creating integrated data systems where all these different kinds of data are linked together. The real problems arise from data quality issues, he continued. "Yes, if you ask the physician to enter more data, you may get more accurate data, but that's going to take the physician away from treating the patient, so that's not necessarily the right approach."

Karen Glanz commented that people go to many different pharmacies, which complicates the collection of data. "I've done studies on glaucoma where we couldn't even get [data on] whether prescriptions were filled," she said, and she suggested that it would be valuable to set up registries to collect this sort of data. It is also very useful, she added, to collect data on patients' social determinants of health—such things as socioeconomic levels and whether patients have housing instability or food insecurity. "It's probably one of the greatest variables where we see a lot of missing data in electronic medical records," she said, "because it's voluntary. It's whether people want to answer, and it's also at a pretty crude level."

Elizabeth Mietlicki-Baase asked if anyone is tracking the outcomes or adverse effects of compounded versions of GLP-1R agonists, which some people have turned to because of the shortages of the manufactured versions. Kosko said that a team at FDA is tracking adverse effects for the compounded versions. Glanz referred to a recently published article (Ashraf et al., 2024) that studied compounding pharmacies that were advertising GLP-1R agonists online and found that most of them did not satisfy all the criteria for compounding pharmacies and at least one was providing drugs that were fake and potentially dangerous.

Peter Park, a clinical scientist at Eli Lilly, asked if there are countries with national health systems that collect good, well-structured data for use in real-world evidence analyses. Bian said that he believes the lack of such structured data is universal "because the documentation burden is huge." Indeed, some Asian countries do not even have electronic health record systems. Thus, it will be important to find ways, perhaps based on artificial intelligence, to extract real-world information from physicians' notes and turn that information into structured data.

Glanz added that another part of the challenges is that physicians' records generally do not even contain much of the information needed for analyses. For instance, many doctors prescribe treatments for patients and ask the patients to let them know if there are any problems, so there may be no record of concerns or successful results. In her use of a GLP-1R agonist, it was the pharmacist who asked her to report any side effects, so those would not be listed in her medical record at the doctor's office.

Prior Authorization and Supply

Stanford commented that one hurdle for patients seeking GLP-1R agonists is prior authorization from insurance companies, which can be quite time-consuming to obtain. Massachusetts General Hospital has a central prior authorization team, and on average each prior authorization for one patient takes 1 hour. "We've seen this year already 51,000 patients at the Mass General Hospital weight center," she said, translating into a tremendous amount of effort spent just on prior authorizations, and it will only get worse once GLP-1R agonists are commonly prescribed for other diseases.

Nicole Boschi, the director of regulatory affairs at the National Multiple Sclerosis Society, pointed out that enabling Medicare and Medicaid to pay for weight loss drugs will require a change in current laws. Stanford said that there is a proposed bill, the Treat and Reduce Obesity Act, which would make that change, but after 12 years of effort, it has still not been passed.[1] Concerning the supply of these drugs, Kosko said that both of the major manufacturers of GLP-1R agonists are working to increase supply by adding manufacturing lines at existing facilities or bringing new facilities online, and the FDA is working to assist them with these expansions. "But we know the demand just continues to increase for these products and will with these new indications," Kosko said.

Health Equity

Guo asked the panelists for strategies for avoiding the growing disparities in the availability of GLP-1R agonists and improving health equity. Stanford suggested that there are lessons to be learned from how the costs of HIV drug regimens were brought down after effective HIV drugs were developed in the late 1990s. This is particularly relevant because people with HIV need to stay on their drugs for life, and it appears that people using GLP-1R agonists for obesity may also need to maintain their usage indefinitely. Bian agreed, noting the PrEP and HIV antiviral drugs are covered by Medicaid.

A workshop participant asked Stanford how the systemic challenges of access to GLP-1R agonists compare between the United States and other countries, such as Canada, that have public health systems. Stanford answered that one difference can be found in the costs of the drugs; for instance, the average monthly price for semaglutide in the United States is about $1,400, while it is $278 in Canada. In other high-income countries around the world, she added, government-negotiated drug prices tend to be significantly lower than in the United States.

In conclusion, one of the themes shared by several workshop participants is that real-world data can play an important role in answering various questions about the use of GLP-1R agonists to treat various disorders;

---

[1] For more information on the Treat and Reduce Obesity Act, see https://www.congress.gov/bill/118th-congress/house-bill/4818 (accessed November 27, 2024).

one valuable way to use the data is in trial emulation. Maximizing the usefulness of such real-world data will, however, require overcoming a number of challenges, such as misclassification issues and varying standards and formats. Workshop participants also highlighted gaps in health care access and quality as another challenge in the field, given that systemically marginalized and under-resourced populations are already finding it more difficult than members of other groups to gain access to GLP-1R agonists to treat obesity.

8

Workshop Reflections and Opportunities to Move Forward

HIGHLIGHTS

- The field of GLP-1R agonists is at an inflection point, where new forms and new uses for this class of medicines are appearing rapidly. But more data are needed to understand the biological mechanisms underpinning the effects of these medications and to understand their risks and benefits in various populations. (Coghlan)
- Studies are needed to understand more about individual differences in response to GLP-1R agonists, and they should take into account patients' genetic, physical, and social characteristics. (Montoya)
- The success of GLP-1R agonists in clinical use will depend in part on encouraging a clear and accurate public understanding of the new drugs. (Glanz)
- The treatment of substance use disorders with GLP-1R agonists will be complicated by the accompanying stigma, similar to what has happened with obesity treatment. (Glanz)
- It would be valuable if academia, the pharmaceutical industry, and government agencies worked together to build integrated datasets with data on mechanisms, omics, biomarkers, imaging, socioeconomic determinants, and clinical measurements

continued

and outcomes. The ultimate goal would be to enable precision medicine using GLP-1R agonists. (Guo)
- The field would benefit from researchers and clinicians understanding the real-world experiences of patients taking GLP-1R agonists, such as how side effects of a drug may influence their lives. (Nece)

NOTE: This list is the rapporteurs' summary of points made by the individual speakers identified, and the statements have not been endorsed or verified by the National Academies of Sciences, Engineering, and Medicine. They are not intended to reflect a consensus among workshop participants.

Matthew Hayes began the final session by commenting that a wide range of perspectives were represented at the workshop, including government, academia, industry, and biotech. "It speaks volumes to me that so many stakeholders are showing interest in the repurposing of GLP-1Rs beyond their current approval for diabetes or obesity," he said. Brian Fiske shared that the speakers in this session would synthesize the main topics from the workshop (see Box 7-1) and hear from a panel of diverse participants about their perception of the field and how it can move forward.

BOX 7-1
Workshop Highlights

- The current promise of GLP-1R agonists in treating a variety of disorders is grounded in three decades of preclinical and clinical research. Today these medicines are approved by the Food and Drug Administration to treat type 2 diabetes and obesity, and they are being tested against a wide variety of other disorders, including central nervous system disorders such as Parkinson's disease and substance use disorders. (Drucker)
- There is both preclinical and clinical evidence that GLP-1R agonists may be effective treatments across a spectrum of central nervous system disorders, including neurodegenerative diseases and substance use disorders, but there is a need for more research and more discussion about clinical trial design, data collection, and real-world evidence analysis. (Athauda, Coghlan, Farokhnia, Greig, Grigson, Jerlhag, McElroy, Mietlicki-Baase, Richardson, Schmidt, Sinclair, Xu)
- GLP-1 receptors are found in multiple places throughout the central nervous system, such as many subcortical areas as well as cortical and hippocampal regions, though not all of these receptors can be accessed by some exog-

continued

> **BOX 7-1 Continued**
>
> enously applied agonists. There are still many unanswered questions about how GLP-1R agonists act in the brain. (Davis, Rinaman)
> - Future research is needed to assess the penetrance of these agonists across the blood–brain barrier, to understand what determines a responder versus nonresponder, the role of biomarkers, and other aspects of the drugs' effectiveness. This research will be most effective as a collaborative effort among academia, industry, government, patient advocacy groups, and patients themselves. (Guo, Hölscher, Jawidzik, Montoya)
> - Real-world data will be vital to advancing the field, and sharing evidence-based information will be important to combat ongoing stigma as these drugs become more widespread. (Bian, Glanz, Guo, Kosko, Nece, Stanford)
> - All of the diseases discussed in the workshop are biologically based and are not a consequence of personal choices. Treatments should be focused on targeting the cause of the symptoms, not just mitigating the symptoms. (Glanz, Leggio, Nece, Richardson, Stanford)
>
> NOTE: This list is the rapporteurs' summary of points made by the individual speakers identified, and the statements have not been endorsed or verified by the National Academies of Sciences, Engineering, and Medicine. They are not intended to reflect a consensus among workshop participants.

PANEL DISCUSSION

An Industry Perspective

Speaking from his perspective as a scientist, Matthew Coghlan said he very much appreciated hearing from Patricia Nece and Karen Glanz, participants with lived experiences. In addition, he spoke of some early experiences in the search for drugs that could treat diabetes and obesity. "I remember almost 20 years ago in one of my early companies, when we had the opportunity to license the original molecule, it was laughed out of the room," he said. "Who would want an injectable?" This was exenatide, with the brand name Byetta, and it was the start of the GLP-1 revolution.

So it is great, he continued, to be in the field now as it experiences an inflection point, where new forms and new uses for this class of medicines are appearing rapidly. "I think it's an exciting time," he said.

"But what I've learned today," he continued, "is we need more data," particularly to understand the biological mechanisms underpinning the drugs' clinical effects. This will help, for example, in determining which preclinical effects are likely to translate into the clinic, said Coghlan.

Finally, he said, the field needs to push forward on the "fantastic opportunities to expand into CNS [central nervous system] disorders and other areas of disease." Coghlan highlighted that this will require preclinical research to point the way to the treatments most likely to be useful in humans and, most important, getting data from clinical trials to determine conclusively which of these new drugs will be safe and effective in humans.

A Government Perspective

Iván Montoya began by offering some background information on the National Institute on Drug Abuse (NIDA) and its Division of Therapeutics and Medical Consequences at the National Institutes of Health, which works with academia and industry to develop medications and other therapeutics for the treatment of substance use disorders. The division supports research—including many of the studies presented at the workshop—through grants and contracts, he said.

Montoya said he was intrigued by the idea of an endogenous GLP-1 system. People in the substance use disorder field are familiar with the endogenous cannabinoid system and the endogenous opioid system, and this is an analogous concept. In particular, he is interested in the development of the GLP-1 system and what factors might shape it.

He drew a distinction between the work now being done with GLP-1R agonists to treat obesity and diabetes, with drugs that have received FDA approval, and the work on treating neuropsychiatric disorders, with drugs that have not. "There is no FDA [Food and Drug Administration] approval for any GLP-1 agonist for substance use disorders," he said. As a result, the data concerning substance use disorders are very preliminary.

The individual differences in the response to GLP-1R agonists was another issue that caught his eye, he said. Although there are not enough data concerning the treatment of substance use disorders to conclusively say much about individual differences, differences in response are evident in the treatment of obesity and diabetes. Studies are needed to understand more about these differences, and they should take into account patients' genetic, physical, and social characteristics, Montoya said.

Noting that one of the objectives of the workshop was to examine the clinical trial and regulatory considerations of GLP-1R agonists, Montoya said that this objective was not well addressed during the meeting. "I think we need to have more discussion about the clinical trial designs," he said. For instance, he said, it is possible that GLP-1R agonists can be used for the treatment of polysubstance abuse—that is, the abuse of multiple substances, which is more prevalent than the abuse of single substances. But what sort of trial design should be used in addressing that question? The typical trial has one medication and one drug of abuse. Testing a GLP-1R agonist against polysubstance abuse would require a different design than usual. The FDA would need to be involved in determining what sort of designs and endpoints would be acceptable to get a GLP-1R agonist approved for such a treatment, he noted.

He closed by reiterating the interest of NIDA in studying GLP-1R agonists. "We hope to continue working with academia and also with industry and the FDA to develop more protocols and to . . . fund research for more GLP-1R agonists for treatment of substance use disorders," he concluded.

A Lived Experience Perspective on Public Understanding and Policy

Karen Glanz's takeaways from the workshop highlighted the importance of public understanding and public policy. These two areas, she said, will play a role in how effective the GLP-1R agonists ultimately become in the overall population. Concerning public understanding, she said, it will be important for the media to get the message out to the public that the new uses for GLP-1R agonists will not be as straightforward as, for example, simply repurposing semaglutide for Parkinson's disease or Alzheimer's disease or substance use disorder. There is already a lot of discussion about these medications in the media, she added, and not all of it is accurate. More generally, Glanz said, public understanding will be crucial in situations where eye-catching research results appear, such as the potential connection between GLP-1R agonists and suicidal ideation; the public will need access to evidence-based information in such cases.

Switching to the topic of stigma, she said that while the workshop had included discussion of stigma in terms of obesity and obesity management treatment, there was little said about the stigma associated with CNS disorders such as substance use disorders, but individuals with those diseases face stigma when they seek treatment for them. For instance, she said, in many U.S. states a pregnant woman who is using illicit substances is treated as a criminal, "so how can she get adequate care?" This is compounded by the fact that many of the women facing this situation have a low socioeconomic status, live in rural areas, and are from underrepresented populations.

Although obesity is now widely understood to be a disease, she said, many people still see it as a moral failing. "I see those issues crossing over into some of the CNS disorders and into this class of drugs," she continued, "and I think there is a lot of work to be done."

A Real-World-Evidence Researcher's Perspective

After first commenting that she agreed with everyone else about how exciting and promising GLP-1R agonists are for treating CNS disorders, Serena Jingchuan Guo cautioned that there are still many unknowns that will require collecting more preclinical data, clinical trial data, and real-world data. "We still do not yet have a complete picture about the safety profiles, the drugs, and the efficacy profiles," she said. This is particularly important, she added, because the new GLP-1 medicines are being hailed as miracle drugs, and they are being considered for treating many conditions even though there are not enough data on the possible consequences of such treatments. But with enough data, researchers and clinicians can do such things as disease phenotyping, identifying the patients most or least likely to benefit from a particular drug or to have safety issues.

Guo called for academia, the pharmaceutical industry, and government agencies to work together to build integrated datasets with data on mechanisms, omics, biomarkers, imaging, socioeconomic determinants, and clinical measurements and outcomes. The ultimate goal would be to enable precision medicine using the GLP-1R agonists.

A Lived Experience Perspective on GLP-1R Progress

Patricia Nece said that she was impressed and excited to hear about all the work going on with GLP-1R agonists. "Most of this is new to me, and it's exciting," she said. "I know people with all these different conditions, and it's so important to come up with adequate and successful treatments for them so that they can just live their lives. Just live their lives—that's all they want to do. . . . And the work you're doing is certainly going to move the needle, I am confident on that score, for these patients."

She did caution, however, that the GLP-1 medicines should not be thought of as miracle drugs. For one thing, not everyone can tolerate them, and results vary from person to person. Furthermore, she added, "it certainly isn't a snap-your-fingers-and-your-obesity-is-gone drug. You have to work at this. Every day I work at it. I wouldn't overpromise as you're developing these new drugs and other therapies."

Nece also said that she was struck by the discussions about teasing apart the different ways in which GLP-1R agonists enact their different effects and the relation between their effects on weight and on other factors, such as cholesterol levels or inflammation. "I think it's fascinating, and I think parsing that out could lead to other discoveries."

Finally, she said, it is vital that researchers and clinicians understand and keep in mind the real-world experiences that patients have, such as how a drug's side effects may influence their lives. "I hope you'll just keep patients in mind with everything you're doing," she said. "It's so easy to get caught up in the minor details. I hope you'll lift your head and look at the bigger picture."

DISCUSSION

The High Prevalence and Cost of Disease in the United States

Mahin Khatami asked why there is a high prevalence of illness in the United States despite the large amount of spending in health care, including for the treatment of cancer, neurodegenerative diseases, and autoimmune diseases.

"It's a great question," Hayes said. Many of these diseases, especially metabolic diseases, have multiple underlying causes and a complex etiology. "And for some of the other CNS diseases we've covered today," he continued, "the complexity just deepens. But it's an important topic to look and consider—not only how we treat the disease, but what perpetuates and causes the disease."

Alexandra Sinclair said that in the United Kingdom decisions about which drugs patients can access take into account considerations from health economics, a topic that had not come up in the workshop. "I wanted just to urge us to think a little bit about building in health economic assessments into our clinical trial design," she said. Then decisions about the drug will consider not only the cost of the drug but also the cost savings resulting from its use.

GLP-1R Agonists in the Pediatric Population and Long-Term Use

Linda Rinaman noted that the FDA has approved some GLP-1R agonists for the treatment of obesity in children as young as 12 years old. She said, "I continue to be amazed that there is so little basic science research, let alone clinical research, about what the effect of that is on the developing brain." How might these drugs change the brains of adolescents and teenagers, and might the changes be permanent? She urged anyone funding or conducting basic science to recognize the importance of these questions. "'I think that we have the tools with the animal models to get at a lot of these questions," she said.

Guo responded that her group is doing a meta-analysis of 17 clinical trials to look at the effects of GLP-1R agonists in the pediatric population, but they do not yet have the results. They are also looking at data from electronic health records from the OneFlorida+ network, which has a large proportion of pediatric patients. And Montoya added that NIDA would be very interested in funding studies exploring how the GLP-1 system develops and how GLP-1R agonists can affect the developing brain.

Chris Brandl from Pennsylvania State University asked about long-term use of GLP-1R agonists. Guo said that there is an ongoing debate about whether patients with obesity will need to take the drugs for the rest of their lives. "We saw some data that when you stopped the medication, you have some regain of weight," she said, "but it seems the weight management is still better than before you took the drug." For semaglutide specifically, which was approved in 2021, there are only 2 to 3 years of clinical data available, "but with time going on we will have more data to answer the questions," she noted.

Considerations for Use of GLP-1R in CNS Disorders

Sinclair said it will be important to consider how GLP-1R agonists will be delivered for use against brain-related disorders, such as Alzheimer's disease or substance use disorders. While the agonists used to treat type 2 diabetes and obesity are typically delivered orally or through intramuscular injections, this may not be the best approach for drugs that need to get into the brain. "Should we be thinking about reformulating the drugs for CNS delivery?" she asked.

Ellen Mowry said that although it had not been discussed at the workshop, multiple sclerosis is another neurodegenerative disease that may be helped by treatment with GLP-1R agonists. Although the younger-age peripheral immune problem of multiple sclerosis has been solved, the neurodegenerative phase of the disease still requires treatments, and her group is planning a trial of a GLP-1R agonist for that purpose, she said.

CLOSING REMARKS

Many workshop participants discussed how both preclinical and clinical data point to the potential for GLP-1R agonists to be effective in treating not only obesity and type 2 diabetes but also various CNS disorders, including ingestive behavior disorders, neurodegenerative diseases, and substance use disorders. However, workshop participants highlighted that questions remain regarding how GLP-1R agonists enter the brain, their mechanisms of action, ensuring fair access to different populations, and evidence-based public education. Throughout the process, researchers, clinicians, policy makers, and drug developers may benefit from considering the perspectives and needs of individuals who could potentially receive GLP-1R agonist.

Appendix A

References

Agüera, Z., M. Lozano-Madrid, N. Mallorquí-Bagué, S. Jiménez-Murcia, J. M. Menchón, and F. Fernández-Aranda. 2021. A review of binge eating disorder and obesity. *Neuropsychiatry* 35(2):57–67.

Allison, K. C., A. M. Chao, M. B. Bruzas, C. McCuen-Wurst, E. Jones, C. McAllister, K. Gruber, R. I. Berkowitz, T. A. Wadden, and J. S. Tronieri. 2022. A pilot randomized controlled trial of liraglutide 3.0 mg for binge eating disorder. *Obesity Science and Practice* 9(2):127–136.

Aoun, L., S. Almardini, F. Saliba, F. Haddadin, O. Mourad, J. Jdaidani, Z. Morcos, I. Al Saidi, E. Bou Sanayeh, S. Saliba, M. Almardini, and J. Zaidan. 2024. GLP-1 receptor agonists: A novel pharmacotherapy for binge eating (binge eating disorder and bulimia nervosa)? A systematic review. *Journal of Clinical & Translational Endocrinology* 35:100333.

Aranäs, C., C. E. Edvardsson, O. T. Shevchouk, Q. Zhang, S. Witley, S. Blid Sköldheden, L. Zentveld, D. Vallöf, M. Tufvesson-Alm, and E. Jerlhag. 2023. Semaglutide reduces alcohol intake and relapse-like drinking in male and female rats. *EBioMedicine* 93:104642.

Aronne, L. J., N. Sattar, D. B. Horn, H. E. Bays, S. Wharton, W.-Y. Lin, N. N. Ahmad, S. Zhang, R. Liao, and M. C. Bunck. 2024. Continued treatment with tirzepatide for maintenance of weight reduction in adults with obesity: The surmount-4 randomized clinical trial. *JAMA* 331(1):38–48.

Ashraf, A. R., T. K. Mackey, J. Schmidt, G. Kulcsár, R. G. Vida, J. Li, and A. Fittler. 2024. Safety and risk assessment of no-prescription online semaglutide purchases. *JAMA Network Open* 7(8):e2428280.

Athauda, D., K. Maclagan, S. S. Skene, M. Bajwa-Joseph, D. Letchford, K. Chowdhury, S. Hibbert, N. Budnik, L. Zampedri, J. Dickson, Y. Li, I. Aviles-Olmos, T. T. Warner, P. Limousin, A. J. Lees, N. H. Greig, S. Tebbs, and T. Foltynie. 2017. Exenatide once weekly versus placebo in Parkinson's disease: A randomised, double-blind, placebo-controlled trial. *The Lancet* 390(10103):1664–1675.

Athauda, D., K. Maclagan, N. Budnik, L. Zampedri, S. Hibbert, S. S. Skene, K. Chowdhury, I. Aviles-Olmos, P. Limousin, and T. Foltynie. 2018. What effects might exenatide have on non-motor symptoms in Parkinson's disease: A post hoc analysis. *Journal of Parkinson's Disease* 8(2):247–258.

Athauda, D., S. Gulyani, H. K. Karnati, Y. Li, D. Tweedie, M. Mustapic, S. Chawla, K. Chowdhury, S. S. Skene, N. H. Greig, D. Kapogiannis, and T. Foltynie. 2019. Utility of neuronal-derived exosomes to examine molecular mechanisms that affect motor function in patients with Parkinson disease: A secondary analysis of the Exenatide-PD Trial. *JAMA Neurology* 76(4):420–429.

Aviles-Olmos, I., J. Dickson, Z. Kefalopoulou, A. Djamshidian, P. Ell, T. Soderlund, P. Whitton, R. Wyse, T. Isaacs, A. Lees, P. Limousin, and T. Foltynie. 2013. Exenatide and the treatment of patients with Parkinson's disease. *Journal of Clinical Investigations* 123(6):2730–2736.

Balantekin, K. N., M. J. Kretz, and E. G. Mietlicki-Baase. 2024. The emerging role of glucagon-like peptide 1 in binge eating. *Journal of Endocrinology* 262(1):e230405.

Barrera, J. G., K. R. Jones, J. P. Herman, D. A. D'Alessio, S. C. Woods, and R. J. Seeley. 2011. Hyperphagia and increased fat accumulation in two models of chronic CNS glucagon-like peptide-1 loss of function. *Journal of Neuroscience* 31(10):3904–3913.

Boileau, I., J. M. Assaad, R. O. Pihl, C. Benkelfat, M. Leyton, M. Diksic, R. E. Tremblay, and A. Dagher. 2003. Alcohol promotes dopamine release in the human nucleus accumbens. *Synapse* 49(4):226–231.

Botfield, H. F., M. S. Uldall, C. S. J. Westgate, J. L. Mitchell, S. M. Hagen, A. M. Gonzalez, D. J. Hodson, R. H. Jensen, and A. J. Sinclair. 2017. A glucagon-like peptide-1 receptor agonist reduces intracranial pressure in a rat model of hydrocephalus. *Science Translational Medicine* 9(404):eaan0972.

Brauer, R., L. Wei, T. Ma, D. Athauda, C. Girges, N. Vijiaratnam, G. Auld, C. Whittlesea, I. Wong, and T. Foltynie. 2020. Diabetes medications and risk of Parkinson's disease: A cohort study of patients with diabetes. *Brain* 143(10):3067–3076.

Brierley, D. I., M. K. Holt, A. Singh, A. de Araujo, M. McDougle, M. Vergara, M. H. Afaghani, S. J. Lee, K. Scott, C. Maske, W. Langhans, E. Krause, A. de Kloet, F. M. Gribble, F. Reimann, L. Rinaman, G. de Lartigue, and S. Trapp. 2021. Central and peripheral GLP-1 systems independently suppress eating. *Nature Metabolism* 3(2):258–273.

Bruns, N., VI, E. H. Tressler, L. F. Vendruscolo, L. Leggio, and M. Farokhnia. 2024. IUPHAR review—Glucagon-like peptide-1 (GLP-1) and substance use disorders: An emerging pharmacotherapeutic target. *Pharmacological Research* 207:107312.

Campbell, J. E., T. D. Müller, B. Finan, R. D. DiMarchi, M. H. Tschöp, and D. A. D'Alessio. 2023. GIPR/GLP-1R dual agonist therapies for diabetes and weight loss—Chemistry, physiology, and clinical applications. *Cell Metabolism* 35(9):1519–1529.

Card, J. P., A. L. Johnson, I. J. Llewellyn-Smith, H. Zheng, R. Anand, D. I. Brierley, S. Trapp, and L. Rinaman. 2018. GLP-1 neurons form a local synaptic circuit within the rodent nucleus of the solitary tract. *Journal of Comparative Neurology* 526(14):2149–2164.

Chang, M. 2022. Despite failing phase 2a clinical trials, Peptron not giving up on Parkinson's treatment. *Korea Biomedical Review*, December 22. https://www.koreabiomed.com/news/articleView.html?idxno=20071 (accessed September 22, 2024).

Chen, W.-H., Y. Li, L. Yang, J. M. Allen, H. Shao, W. T. Donahoo, L. Billelo, X. Hu, E. A. Shenkman, and J. Bian. 2024. Geographic variation and racial disparities in adoption of newer glucose-lowering drugs with cardiovascular benefits among US Medicare beneficiaries with type 2 diabetes. *Plos One* 19(1):e0297208.

Christensen, M., A. H. Sparre-Ulrich, B. Hartmann, U. Grevstad, M. M. Rosenkilde, J. J. Holst, T. Vilsbøll, and F. K. Knop. 2015. Transfer of liraglutide from blood to cerebrospinal fluid is minimal in patients with type 2 diabetes. *International Journal of Obesity (London)* 39(11):1651–1654.

Chuong, V., M. Farokhnia, S. Khom, C. L. Pince, S. K. Elvig, R. Vlkolinsky, R. C. Marchette, G. F. Koob, M. Roberto, L. F. Vendruscolo, and L. Leggio. 2023. The glucagon-like peptide-1 (GLP-1) analogue semaglutide reduces alcohol drinking and modulates central GABA neurotransmission. *JCI Insight* 8(12):e170671.

Cleveland, H. H., K. S. Knapp, T. R. Brick, M. A. Russell, J. M. Gajos, and S. C. Bunce. 2021. Effectiveness and utility of mobile device assessment of subjective craving during residential opioid dependence treatment. *Substance Use & Misuse* 56(9):1284–1294.

Collins, L., and R. A. Costello. 2019. *Glucagon-like peptide-1 receptor agonists*. Treasure Island, FL: StatPearls. https://www.ncbi.nlm.nih.gov/books/NBK551568/ (accessed November 27, 2024).

Concato, J., and J. Corrigan-Curay. 2022. Real-world evidence—Where are we now? *New England Journal of Medicine* 386(18):1680–1682.

Deloitte Access Economics. 2020. *The social and economic cost of eating disorders in the United States of America: A report for the Strategic Training Initiative for the Prevention of Eating Disorders and the Academy for Eating Disorders*. Available at: https://www.hsph.harvard.edu/striped/report-economic-costs-of-eating-disorders/ (accessed September 26, 2024).

Doucleff, M. 2023. Ozempic seems to curb cravings for alcohol. Here's what scientists think is going on. *NPR News*, August 28. https://www.npr.org/sections/health-shots/2023/08/28/1194526119/ozempic-wegovy-drinking-alcohol-cravings-semaglutide (accessed October 1, 2024).

Douton, J. E., N. K. Acharya, B. Stoltzfus, D. Sun, P. S. Grigson, and J. E. Nyland. 2022. Acute glucagon-like peptide-1 receptor agonist liraglutide prevents cue-, stress-, and drug-induced heroin-seeking in rats. *Behavioral Pharmacology* 33(5):364–378.

Drucker, D. J. 2022. GLP-1 physiology informs the pharmacotherapy of obesity. *Molecular Metabolism* 57:101351.

Drucker, D. J. 2024. The benefits of GLP-1 drugs beyond obesity. *Science* 385(6706):258–260.

Drucker, D. J., and J. J. Holst. 2023. The expanding incretin universe: From basic biology to clinical translation. *Diabetologia* 66(10):1765–1779.

Drucker, D. J., J. Philippe, S. Mojsov, W. L. Chick, and J. F. Habener. 1987. Glucagon-like peptide 1 stimulates insulin gene expression and increases cyclic amp levels in a rat islet cell line. *Proceedings of the National Academy of Sciences* 84(10):3434–3438.

During, M. J., L. Cao, D. S. Zuzga, J. S. Francis, H. L. Fitzsimons, X. Jiao, R. J. Bland, M. Klugmann, W. A. Banks, and D. J. Drucker. 2003. Glucagon-like peptide-1 receptor is involved in learning and neuroprotection. *Nature Medicine* 9(9):1173–1179.

Egecioglu, E., P. Steensland, I. Fredriksson, K. Feltmann, J. A. Engel, and E. Jerlhag. 2013. The glucagon-like peptide 1 analogue exendin-4 attenuates alcohol mediated behaviors in rodents. *Psychoneuroendocrinology* 38(8):1259–1270.

Evans, B., B. Stoltzfus, N. Acharya, J. E. Nyland, A. C. Arnold, C. S. Freet, S. C. Bunce, and P. S. Grigson. 2022. Dose titration with the glucagon-like peptide 1 agonist, liraglutide, reduces cue- and drug-induced heroin seeking in high drug-taking rats. *Brain Research Bulletin* 189:163–173.

Fang, J., P. Miller, and P. S. Grigson. 2023. Sleep is increased by liraglutide, a glucagon-like peptide-1 receptor agonist, in rats. *Brain Research Bulletin* 192:142–155.

Farkas, E., A. Szilvásy-Szabó, Y. Ruska, R. Sinkó, M. G. Rasch, T. Egebjerg, C. Pyke, B. Gereben, L. B. Knudsen, and C. Fekete. 2021. Distribution and ultrastructural localization of the glucagon-like peptide-1 receptor (GLP-1R) in the rat brain. *Brain Structure and Function* 226(1):225–245.

FDA-NIH (Food and Drug Administration and National Institutes of Health) Biomarker Working Group. n.d. *BEST (Biomarkers, EndpointS, and other Tools) Resource*. Silver Spring, MD: Food and Drug Administration. https://www.ncbi.nlm.nih.gov/books/NBK326791/ (accessed September 22, 2024).

Femminella, G. D., E. Frangou, S. B. Love, G. Busza, C. Holmes, C. Ritchie, R. Lawrence, B. McFarlane, G. Tadros, B. H. Ridha, C. Bannister, Z. Walker, H. Archer, E. Coulthard, B. R. Underwood, A. Prasanna, P. Koranteng, S. Karim, K. Junaid, B. McGuinness, R. Nilforooshan, A. Macharouthu, A. Donaldson, S. Thacker, G. Russell, N. Malik, V. Mate, L. Knight, S. Kshemendran, J. Harrison, C. Hölscher, D. J. Brooks, A. P. Passmore, C. Ballard, and P. Edison. 2019. Evaluating the effects of the novel GLP-1 analogue liraglutide in Alzheimer's disease: Study protocol for a randomised controlled trial (ELAD study). *Trials* 20(1):191.

Feng, P., X. Zhang, D. Li, C. Ji, Z. Yuan, R. Wang, G. Xue, G. Li, and C. Hölscher. 2018. Two novel dual GLP-1/GIP receptor agonists are neuroprotective in the MPTP mouse model of Parkinson's disease. *Neuropharmacology* 133:385–394.

Gabery, S., C. G. Salinas, S. J. Paulsen, J. Ahnfelt-Rønne, T. Alanentalo, A. F. Baquero, S. T. Buckley, E. Farkas, C. Fekete, K. S. Frederiksen, H. C. C. Helms, J. F. Jeppesen, L. M. John, C. Pyke, J. Nøhr, T. T. Lu, J. Polex-Wolf, V. Prevot, K. Raun, L. Simonsen, G. Sun, A. Szilvásy-Szabó, H. Willenbrock, A. Secher, L. B. Knudsen, and W. F. J. Hogendorf. 2020. Semaglutide lowers body weight in rodents via distributed neural pathways. *JCI Insight* 5(6):e133429.

Garvey, W. T., J. I. Mechanick, E. M. Brett, A. J. Garber, D. L. Hurley, A. M. Jastreboff, K. Nadolsky, R. Pessah-Pollack, and R. Plodkowski. 2016. American Association of Clinical Endocrinologists and American College of Endocrinology comprehensive clinical practice guidelines for medical care of patients with obesity. *Endocrine Practice* 22(Suppl 3):1–203.

Glanz, K., J. F. Sallis, B. E. Saelens, and L. D. Frank. 2005. Healthy nutrition environments: Concepts and measures. *American Journal of Health Promotion* 19(5):330–333, ii.

Glanz, K., S. Murphy, J. Moylan, D. Evensen, and J. D. Curb. 2006. Improving dietary self-monitoring and adherence with hand-held computers: A pilot study. *American Journal of Health Promotion* 20(3):165–170.

Glanz, K., P. A. Shaw, P. L Kwong, J. R. Choi, A. Chung, J. Zhu, Q. E. Huang, K. Hoffer, and K. G. Volpp. 2021. Effect of financial incentives and environmental strategies on weight loss in the Healthy Weigh Study: A randomized clinical trial. *JAMA Network Open* 4(9):e2124132.

Glanz, K., A. K. Fultz, J. F. Sallis, M. Clawson, K. C. McLaughlin, S. Green, and B. E. Saelens. 2023. Use of the Nutrition Environment Measures Survey: A systematic review. *American Journal of Preventive Medicine* 65(1):131–142.

Gu, G., B. Roland, K. Tomaselli, C. S. Dolman, C. Lowe, and J. S. Heilig. 2013. Glucagon-like peptide-1 in the rat brain: Distribution of expression and functional implication. *Journal of Comparative Neurology* 521(10):2235–2261.

Hallaj, S., W. Halfpenny, B. G. Chuter, R. N. Weinreb, S. L. Baxter, Q. N. Cui. 2025. Association between glucagon-like peptide 1 (GLP-1) receptor agonists exposure and intraocular pressure change. *American Journal of Ophthalmology* 269:255–265. https://doi.org/10.1016/j.ajo.2024.08.030.

Halloum, W., Y. A. Dughem, D. Beier, and L. Pellesi. 2024. Glucagon-like peptide-1 (GLP-1) receptor agonists for headache and pain disorders: A systematic review. *Journal of Headache and Pain* 25(1):112.

Heilig, M., J. MacKillop, D. Martinez, J. Rehm, L. Leggio, and L. J. M. J. Vanderschuren. 2021. Addiction as a brain disease revised: Why it still matters, and the need for consilience. *Neuropsychopharmacology* 46:1715–1723.

Hernandez, N. S., and H. D. Schmidt. 2019. Central GLP-1 receptors: Novel molecular targets for cocaine use disorder. *Physiology & Behavior* 206:93–105.

Hernandez, N. S., K. Y. Ige, E. G. Mietlicki-Baase, G. C. Molina-Castro, C. A. Turner, M. R. Hayes, and H. D. Schmidt. 2018. Glucagon-like peptide-1 receptor activation in the ventral tegmental area attenuates cocaine seeking in rats. *Neuropsychopharmacology* 43(10):2000–2008.

Hernandez, N. S., V. R. Weir, K. Ragnini, R. Merkel, Y. Zhang, K. Mace, M. T. Rich, R. Christopher Pierce, and H. D. Schmidt. 2021. GLP-1 receptor signaling in the laterodorsal tegmental nucleus attenuates cocaine seeking by activating GABAergic circuits that project to the VTA. *Molecular Psychiatry* 26(8):4394–4408.

Hinnen, D. 2017. Glucagon-like peptide 1 receptor agonists for type 2 diabetes. *Diabetes Spectrum* 30(3):202–210.

Hölscher, C. 2022. Protective properties of GLP-1 and associated peptide hormones in neurodegenerative disorders. *British Journal of Pharmacology* 179(4):695–714.

Holt, M. K., J. E. Richards, D. R. Cook, D. I. Brierley, D. L. Williams, F. Reimann, F. M. Gribble, and S. Trapp. 2019. Preproglucagon neurons in the nucleus of the solitary tract are the main source of brain GLP-1, mediate stress-induced hypophagia, and limit unusually large intakes of food. *Diabetes* 68(1):21–33.

Huang, K. P., A. A. Acosta, M. Y. Ghidewon, A. D. McKnight, M. S. Almeida, N. T. Nyema, N. D. Hanchak, N. Patel, Y. S. K. Gbenou, A. E. Adriaenssens, K. A. Bolding, and A. L. Alhadeff. 2024. Dissociable hindbrain GLP1R circuits for satiety and aversion. *Nature* 632(8025):585–593.

Hudson, J. I., E. Hiripi, H. G. Pope Jr., and R. C. Kessler. 2007. The prevalence and correlates of eating disorders in the National Comorbidity Survey Replication. *Biological Psychiatry* 61(3):348–358. Erratum in: *Biological Psychiatry* 72(2):164.

Jastreboff, A. M., L. J. Aronne, N. N. Ahmad, S. Wharton, L. Connery, B. Alves, A. Kiyosue, S. Zhang, B. Liu, and M. C. Bunck. 2022. Tirzepatide once weekly for the treatment of obesity. *New England Journal of Medicine* 387(3):205–216.

Jerlhag, E. 2023. The therapeutic potential of glucagon-like peptide-1 for persons with addictions based on findings from preclinical and clinical studies. *Frontiers in Pharmacology* 14:1063033.

Jia, Y., N. Gong, T.-F. Li, B. Zhu, and Y.-X. Wang. 2015. Peptidic exenatide and herbal catalpol mediate neuroprotection via the hippocampal GLP-1 receptor/β-endorphin pathway. *Pharmacological Research* 102:276–285.

Jing, F., Q. Zou, Y. Wang, Z. Cai, and Y. Tang. 2021. Activation of microglial GLP-1R in the trigeminal nucleus caudalis suppresses central sensitization of chronic migraine after recurrent nitroglycerin stimulation. *Journal of Headache and Pain* 22(1):86.

Jing, F., Q. Zou, and Y. Pu. 2023. GLP-1R agonist liraglutide attenuates pain hypersensitivity by stimulating IL-10 release in a nitroglycerin-induced chronic migraine mouse model. *Neuroscience Letters* 812:137397.

Johnson, A. 2024. Increasing evidence suggests Ozempic (semaglutide) helps curb alcoholism. *Forbes*, June 5. https://www.forbes.com/sites/ariannajohnson/2024/06/05/increasing-evidence-suggests-ozempic-semaglutide-helps-curb-alcoholism/ (accessed October 2, 2024).

King, A., A. Vena, D. S. Hasin, D. DeWit, S. J. O'Connor, and D. Cao. 2021. Subjective responses to alcohol in the development and maintenance of alcohol use disorder. *American Journal of Psychiatry* 178(6):560–571.

Klausen, M. K., M. E. Jensen, M. Møller, N. Le Dous, A. Ø. Jensen, V. A. Zeeman, C. F. Johannsen, A. Lee, G. K. Thomsen, J. Macoveanu, P. M. Fisher, M. P. Gillum, N. R. Jørgensen, M. L. Bergmann, H. Enghusen Poulsen, U. Becker, J. J. Holst, H. Benveniste, N. D. Volkow, S. Vollstädt-Klein, K. W. Miskowiak, C. T. Ekstrøm, G. M. Knudsen, T. Vilsbøll, and A. Fink-Jensen. 2022. Exenatide once weekly for alcohol use disorder investigated in a randomized, placebo-controlled clinical trial. *JCI Insight* 7(19):e159863.

Konanur, V. R., T. M. Hsu, S. E. Kanoski, M. R. Hayes, and M. R. Roitman. 2020. Phasic dopamine responses to a food-predictive cue are suppressed by the glucagon-like peptide-1 receptor agonist exendin-4. *Physiology & Behavior* 215:112771.

Kooij, K. L., D. I. Koster, E. Eeltink, M. Luijendijk, L. Drost, F. Ducrocq, and R. A.H. Adan. 2024. GLP-1 receptor agonist semaglutide reduces appetite while increasing dopamine reward signaling. *Neuroscience Applied* 3:103925.

Kopp, K. O., E. J. Glotfelty, Y. Li, and N. H. Greig. 2022. Glucagon-like peptide-1 (GLP-1) receptor agonists and neuroinflammation: Implications for neurodegenerative disease treatment. *Pharmacological Research* 186:106550.

Kopp, K. O., E. J. Glotfelty, Y. Li, D. K. Lahiri, and N. H. Greig. 2024. Type 2 diabetes mellitus/obesity drugs: A neurodegenerative disorders savior or a bridge too far? *Ageing Research Reviews* 98:102343.

Krajnc, N., B. Itariu, S. Macher, W. Marik, J. Harreiter, M. Michl, K. Novak, C. Wöber, B. Pemp, and G. Bsteh. 2023. Treatment with GLP-1 receptor agonists is associated with significant weight loss and favorable headache outcomes in idiopathic intracranial hypertension. *Journal of Headache and Pain* 24(1):89.

Lawrence, E. C. N., M. Guo, T. D. Schwartz, J. Wu, J. Lu, S. Nikonov, J. K. Sterling, and Q. N. Cui. 2023. Topical and systemic GLP-1R agonist administration both rescue retinal ganglion cells in hypertensive glaucoma. *Frontiers in Cellular Neuroscience* 17:1156829.

Leggio, L., C. S. Hendershot, M. Farokhnia, A. Fink-Jensen, M. K. Klausen, J. P. Schacht, and W. K. Simmons. 2023. GLP-1 receptor agonists are promising but unproven treatments for alcohol and substance use disorders. *Nature Medicine* 29(12):2993–2995.

Leshner, A. I. 1997. Addiction is a brain disease, and it matters. *Science* 278(5335):45–47.

Leslie, M. 2023. Hot weight loss drugs tested against addiction. *Science* 381(6661):930–931.

Li, Y., T. Perry, M. S. Kindy, B. K. Harvey, D. Tweedie, H. W. Holloway, K. Powers, H. Shen, J. M. Egan, K. Sambamurti, A. Brossi, D. K. Lahiri, M. P. Mattson, B. J. Hoffer, Y. Wang, and N. H. Greig. 2009. GLP-1 receptor stimulation preserves primary cortical and dopaminergic neurons in cellular and rodent models of stroke and Parkinsonism. *Proceedings of the National Academies of Sciences* 106:1285–1290.

Lincoff, A. M., K. Brown-Frandsen, H. M. Colhoun, J. Deanfield, S. S. Emerson, S. Esbjerg, S. Hardt-Lindberg, G. K. Hovingh, S. E. Kahn, and R. F. Kushner. 2023. Semaglutide and cardiovascular outcomes in obesity without diabetes. *New England Journal of Medicine* 389(24):2221–2232.

Love, A., D. James, and P. Willner. 1998. A comparison of two alcohol craving questionnaires. *Addiction* 93(7):1091–1102.

Lu, Z., N. Percie Du Sert, S. W. Chan, C. K. Yeung, G. Lin, D. T. Yew, P. L. Andrews, and J. A. Rudd. 2014. Differential hypoglycaemic, anorectic, autonomic and emetic effects of the glucagon-like peptide receptor agonist, exendin-4, in the conscious telemetered ferret. *Journal of Translational Medicine* 12:327.

Malatt, C., T. Wu, C. Bresee, E. J. Hogg, J. C. Wertheimer, E. Tan, H. Pomeroy, G. Obialisi, and M. Tagliati. 2022. Liraglutide improves non-motor function and activities of daily living in patients with Parkinson's disease: A randomized, double-blind, placebo-controlled trial. *Neurology* 98(18 Suppl.):3068.

Maniscalco, J. W., and L. Rinaman. 2018. Vagal interoceptive modulation of motivated behavior. *Physiology (Bethesda)* 33(2):151–167.

McClean, P. L., V. Parthsarathy, E. Faivre, and C. Hölscher. 2011. The diabetes drug liraglutide prevents degenerative processes in a mouse model of Alzheimer's disease. *Journal of Neuroscience* 31(17):6587–6594.

McElroy, S. L., A. I. Guerdjikova, N. Mori, and A. M. O'Melia. 2012. Pharmacological management of binge eating disorder: Current and emerging treatment options. *Therapeutics and Clinical Risk Management* 8:219–241.

McElroy, S. L., S. J. Winham, A. B. Cuellar-Barboza, C. L. Colby, A. M. Ho, H. Sicotte, B. R. Larrabee, S. Crow, M. A. Frye, and J. M. Biernacka. 2018. Bipolar disorder with binge eating behavior: A genome-wide association study implicates PRR5-ARHGAP8. *Translational Psychiatry* 8(1):40.

McElroy, S. L., A. I. Guerdjikova, T. J. Blom, N. Mori, and F. Romo-Nava. 2024. Liraglutide in obese or overweight individuals with stable bipolar disorder. *Journal of Clinical Psychopharmacology* 44(2):89–95.

McGarry, A., S. Rosanbalm, M. Leinonen, C. W. Olanow, D. To, A. Bell, D. Lee, J. Chang, J. Dubow, R. Dhall, D. Burdick, S. Parashos, J. Feuerstein, J. Quinn, R. Pahwa, M. Afshari, A. Ramirez-Zamora, K. Chou, A. Tarakad, C. Luca, K. Klos, Y. Bordelon, M. H. St Hiliare, D. Shprecher, S. Lee, T. M. Dawson, V. Roschke, and K. Kieburtz. 2024. Safety, tolerability, and efficacy of NLY01 in early untreated Parkinson's disease: A randomised, double-blind, placebo-controlled trial. *The Lancet Neurology* 23(1):37–45.

Meissner, W. G., P Remy, C. Giordana, D. Maltête, P. Derkinderen, J. L. Houéto, M. Anheim, I. Benatru, T. Boraud, C. Brefel-Courbon, N. Carrière, H. Catala, O. Colin, J. C. Corvol, P. Damier, E. Dellapina, D. Devos, S. Drapier, M. Fabbri, V. Ferrier, A. Foubert-Samier, S. Frismand-Kryloff, A. Georget, C. Germain, S. Grimaldi, C. Hardy, L. Hopes, P. Krystkowiak, B. Laurens, R. Lefaucheur, L. L. Mariani, A. Marques, C. Marse, F. Ory-Magne, V. Rigalleau, H. Salhi, A. Saubion, S. R. W. Stott, C. Thalamas, C. Thiriez, M. Tir, R. K. Wyse, A. Benard, O. Rascol; and the LIXIPARK Study Group. 2024. Trial of lixisenatide in early Parkinson's disease. *New England Journal of Medicine* 390(13):1176–1185.

Mietlicki-Baase, E. G, P. I. Ortinski, L. E. Rupprecht, D. R. Olivos, A. L. Alhadeff, R. C. Pierce, and M. R. Hayes. 2013. The food intake-suppressive effects of glucagon-like peptide-1 receptor signaling in the ventral tegmental area are mediated by AMPA/kainate receptors. *American Journal of Physiology–Endocrinology and Metabolism* 305(11):E1367–E1374.

Mitchell, J. L., H. S. Lyons, J. K. Walker, A. Yiangou, O. Grech, Z. Alimajstorovic, N. H. Greig, Y. Li, G. Tsermoulas, K. Brock, S. P. Mollan, and A. J. Sinclair. 2023. The effect of GLP-1RA exenatide on idiopathic intracranial hypertension: A randomized clinical trial. *Brain* 146(5):1821–1830.

Mukherjee, A., A. Hum, T. J. Gustafson, and E. G. Mietlicki-Baase. 2020. Binge-like palatable food intake in rats reduces preproglucagon in the nucleus tractus solitarius. *Physiology & Behavior* 219:112830.

Müller, T. D., B. Finan, S. Bloom, D. D'Alessio, D. J. Drucker, P. Flatt, A. Fritsche, F. Gribble, H. Grill, and J. Habener. 2019. Glucagon-like peptide 1 (GLP-1). *Molecular Metabolism* 30:72–130.

Niazi, S., F. Gnesin, A. S. Thein, J. R. Andreasen, A. Horwitz, Z. A. Mouhammad, B. N. Jawad, Z. Niazi, N. Pourhadi, B. Zareini, A. Meaidi, C. Torp-Pedersen, and M. Kolko. 2024. Association between glucagon-like peptide-1 receptor agonists and the risk of glaucoma in individuals with type 2 diabetes. *Ophthalmology* 131(9):1056–1063.

Randolph, A. B., H. Zheng, and L. Rinaman. 2024. Populations of hindbrain glucagon-like peptide 1 (GLP1) neurons that innervate the hypothalamic PVH, thalamic PVT, or limbic forebrain BST have axon collaterals that reach all central regions innervated by GLP1 neurons. *Journal of Neuroscience* 44(31):e2063232024.

Resnick, B. 2024. Is Ozempic an anti-desire drug? *Vox*, May 7. https://www.vox.com/science/24086968/glp-1-ozempic-semaglutide-craving-desire-science-wanting-liking-opioids-alcohol (accessed October 2, 2024).

Rhea, E. M., A. Babin, P. Thomas, M. Omer, R. Weaver, K. Hansen, W. A. Banks, and K. Talbot. 2023. Brain uptake pharmacokinetics of albiglutide, dulaglutide, tirzepatide, and DA5-CH in the search for new treatments of Alzheimer's and Parkinson's diseases. *Tissue Barriers*, December 14. https://doi.org/10.1080/21688370.2023.2292461.

Richard, J. E., R. H. Anderberg, L. López-Ferreras, K. Olandersson, and K. P. Skibicka. 2016. Sex and estrogens alter the action of glucagon-like peptide-1 on reward. *Biology of Sex Differences* 7:1–16.

Robert, S. A., A. G. Rohana, S. A. Shah, K. Chinna, W. N. Wan Mohamud, and N. A. Kamaruddin. 2015. Improvement in binge eating in non-diabetic obese individuals after 3 months of treatment with liraglutide—A pilot study. *Obesity Research & Clinical Practice* 9(3):301–304.

Ryan, D. H., I. Lingvay, J. Deanfield, S. E. Kahn, E. Barros, B. Burguera, H. M. Colhoun, C. Cercato, D. Dicker, and D. B. Horn. 2024. Long-term weight loss effects of semaglutide in obesity without diabetes in the SELECT trial. *Nature Medicine* 30:2049–2057.

Salameh, T. S., E. M. Rhea, K. Talbot, and W. A. Banks. 2020. Brain uptake pharmacokinetics of incretin receptor agonists showing promise as Alzheimer's and Parkinson's disease therapeutics. *Biochemical Pharmacology* 180:114187.

Sallis, J. F., and K. Glanz. 2009. Physical activity and food environments: Solutions to the obesity epidemic. *Milbank Quarterly* 87(1):123–154.

Scrocchi, L., T. Brown, N. MaClusky, P. Brubaker, A. Auerbach, A. Joyner, and D. Drucker. 1996. Glucose intolerance but normal satiety in mice with a null mutation in the glucagon-like peptide 1 receptor gene. *Nature Medicine* 2(11):1254–1258.

Secher, A., J. Jelsing, A. F. Baquero, J. Hecksher-Sørensen, M. A. Cowley, L. S. Dalbøge, G. Hansen, K. L. Grove, C. Pyke, K. Raun, L. Schäffer, M. Tang-Christensen, S. Verma, B. M. Witgen, N. Vrang, and L. Bjerre Knudsen. 2014. The arcuate nucleus mediates GLP-1 receptor agonist liraglutide-dependent weight loss. *Journal of Clinical Investigation* 124(10):4473–4488.

Sherman, R. E., S. A. Anderson, G. J. Dal Pan, G. W. Gray, T. Gross, N. L. Hunter, L. LaVange, D. Marinac-Dabic, P. W. Marks, M. A. Robb, J. Shuren, R. Temple, J. Woodcock, L. Q. Yue, and R. M. Califf. 2016. Real-world evidence—What is it and what can it tell us? *New England Journal of Medicine* 375(23):2293–2297.

Sterling, J. K., M. O. Adetunji, S. Guttha, A. R. Bargoud, K. E. Uyhazi, A. G. Ross, J. L. Dunaief, and Q. N. Cui. 2020. GLP-1 receptor agonist NLY01 reduces retinal inflammation and neuron death secondary to ocular hypertension. *Cell Reports* 33(5):108271.

Sterling, J., P. Hua, J. L. Dunaief, Q. N. Cui, and B. L. VanderBeek. 2023. Glucagon-like peptide 1 receptor agonist use is associated with reduced risk for glaucoma. *British Journal of Ophthalmology* 107(2):215–220.

Strain, W. D., O. Frenkel, M. A. James, L. A. Leiter, S. Rasmussen, P. M. Rothwell, M. S. Ripa, T. C. Truelsen, and M. Husain. 2022. Effects of semaglutide on stroke subtypes in type 2 diabetes: Post hoc analysis of the randomized sustain 6 and pioneer 6. *Stroke* 53(9):2749–2757.

Svenningsson, P., K. Wirdefeldt, L. Yin, F. Fang, I. Markaki, S. Efendic, and J. F. Ludvigsson. 2016. Reduced incidence of Parkinson's disease after dipeptidyl peptidase-4 inhibitors—A nationwide case-control study. *Movement Disorders* 31(9):1422–1423.

Tang, H., Y. Lu, M. S. Okun, W. T. Donahoo, A. Ramirez-Zamora, F. Wang, Y. Huang, M. Armstrong, M. Svensson, B. A. Virnig, S. T. DeKosky, J. Bian, and J. Guo. 2024. Glucagon-like peptide-1 receptor agonists and risk of Parkinson's disease in patients with type 2 diabetes: A population-based cohort study. *Movement Disorders* 39(11):1960–1970. https://doi.org/10.1002/mds.29992.

Tang-Christensen, M., P. Larsen, R. Goke, A. Fink-Jensen, D. Jessop, M. Møller, and S. Sheikh. 1996. Central administration of GLP-1-(7-36) amide inhibits food and water intake in rats. *American Journal of Physiology-Regulatory, Integrative and Comparative Physiology* 271(4):R848–R856.

Tirrell, M. 2023. Weight-loss meds like Ozempic may help curb addictive behaviors, but drugmakers aren't running trials to find out. *CNN Health*, June 1. https://www.cnn.com/2023/06/01/health/weight-loss-drugs-addictive-behaviors/ (accessed October 1, 2024).
Tuesta, L. M., Z. Chen, A. Duncan, C. D. Fowler, M. Ishikawa, B. R. Lee, X.-A. Liu, Q. Lu, M. Cameron, and M. R. Hayes. 2017. GLP-1 acts on habenular avoidance circuits to control nicotine intake. *Nature Neuroscience* 20(5):708–716.
Turton, M., D. O'Shea, I. Gunn, S. Beak, C. Edwards, K. Meeran, S. Choi, G. Taylor, M. Heath, and P. Lambert. 1996. A role for glucagon-like peptide-1 in the central regulation of feeding. *Nature* 379(6560):69–72.
Udo, T., and C. M. Grilo. 2018. Prevalence and correlates of DSM-5-defined eating disorders in a nationally representative sample of U.S. adults. *Biological Psychiatry* 84(5):345–354.
Urbanik, L. A., N. K. Acharya, and P. S. Grigson. 2022. Acute treatment with the glucagon-like peptide-1 receptor agonist, liraglutide, reduces cue- and drug-induced fentanyl seeking in rats. *Brain Research Bulletin* 189:155–162.
Urbanik, L. A., J. L. Booth, N. K. Acharya, B. B. Evans, and P. S. Grigson. 2025. Effect of acute treatment with the glucagon-like peptide-1 receptor agonist, liraglutide, and estrus phase on cue- and drug-induced fentanyl seeking in female rats. *Behavioural Pharmacology* 36(1):16–29.
Vallöf, D., P. Maccioni, G. Colombo, M. Mandrapa, J. W. Jörnulf, E. Egecioglu, J. A. Engel, and E. Jerlhag. 2016. The glucagon-like peptide 1 receptor agonist liraglutide attenuates the reinforcing properties of alcohol in rodents. *Addiction Biology* 21(2):422–437.
Vallöf, D., J. Vestlund, and E. Jerlhag. 2019. Glucagon-like peptide-1 receptors within the nucleus of the solitary tract regulate alcohol-mediated behaviors in rodents. *Neuropharmacology* 149:124–132.
Vallöf, D., A. L. Kalafateli, and E. Jerlhag. 2020. Long-term treatment with a glucagon-like peptide-1 receptor agonist reduces ethanol intake in male and female rats. *Translational Psychiatry* 10(1):238.
Villarejo, C., F. Fernández-Aranda, S. Jiménez-Murcia, E. Peñas-Lledó, F. Granero, E. Penelo, F. J. Tinahones, C. Sancho, N. Vilarrasa, M. Montserrat-Gil de Bernabé, F. F. Casanueva, J. M. Fernández-Real, G. Frühbeck, R. De la Torre, J. Treasure, C. Botella, and J. M. Menchón. 2012. Lifetime obesity in patients with eating disorders: Increasing prevalence, clinical and personality correlates. *European Eating Disorders Review* 20(3):250–254.
Volkow, N. D., G. F. Koob, and A. T. McLellan. 2016. Neurobiologic advances from the brain disease model of addiction. *New England Journal of Medicine* 374(4):363–371.
Wadden, T. A., A. M. Chao, S. Machineni, R. Kushner, J. Ard, G. Srivastava, B. Halpern, S. Zhang, J. Chen, and M. C. Bunck. 2023. Tirzepatide after intensive lifestyle intervention in adults with overweight or obesity: The surmount-3 phase 3 trial. *Nature Medicine* 29(11):2909–2918.
Waldrop, S. W., V. R. Johnson, and F. C. Stanford. 2024. Inequalities in the provision of GLP-1 receptor agonists for the treatment of obesity. *Nature Medicine* 30(1):22–25.
Wang, V., T. T. Kuo, E. Y. Huang, K. H. Ma, Y. C. Chou, Z. Y. Fu, L. W. Lai, J. Jung, H. I. Choi, D. S. Choi, Y. Li, L. Olson, N. H. Greig, B. J. Hoffer, and Y. H. Chen. 2021. Sustained release GLP-1 agonist PT320 delays disease progression in a mouse model of Parkinson's disease. *ACS Pharmacology & Translational Science* 4(2):858–869.
Wang, W., N. D. Volkow, N. A. Berger, P. B. Davis, D. C. Kaelber, and R. Xu. 2024a. Associations of semaglutide with incidence and recurrence of alcohol use disorder in real-world population. *Nature Communications* 15:4548.
Wang, W., N. D. Volkow, N. A. Berger, P. B. Davis, D. C. Kaelber, and R. Xu. 2024b. Association of semaglutide with reduced incidence and relapse of cannabis use disorder in real-world populations: A retrospective cohort study. *Molecular Psychiatry* 29(8):2587–2598.

Wang, W., N. D. Volkow, N. A. Berger, P. B. Davis, D. C. Kaelber, and R. Xu. 2024c. Association of semaglutide with tobacco use disorder in patients with type 2 diabetes: Target trial emulation using real-world data. *Annals of Internal Medicine* 177(8):1016–1027.

Wang, W., N. D. Volkow, Q. Wang, N. A. Berger, P. B. Davis, D. C. Kaelber, and R. Xu. 2024d. Semaglutide and opioid overdose risk in patients with type 2 diabetes and opioid use disorder. *JAMA Network Open* 7(9):e2435247.

Wang, W., N. D. Volkow, N. A. Berger, P. B. Davis, D. C. Kaelber, and R. Xu. 2024e. Association of semaglutide with risk of suicidal ideation in a real-world cohort. *Nature Medicine* 30:168–176.

Wilding, J. P., R. L. Batterham, M. Davies, L. F. Van Gaal, K. Kandler, K. Konakli, I. Lingvay, B. M. McGowan, T. K. Oral, and J. Rosenstock. 2022. Weight regain and cardiometabolic effects after withdrawal of semaglutide: The step 1 trial extension. *Diabetes, Obesity and Metabolism* 24(8):1553–1564.

Wong, C. K., B. A. McLean, L. L. Baggio, J. A. Koehler, R. Hammoud, N. Rittig, J. M. Yabut, R. J. Seeley, T. J. Brown, and D. J. Drucker. 2024. Central glucagon-like peptide 1 receptor activation inhibits toll-like receptor agonist-induced inflammation. *Cell Metabolism* 36(1):130–143. e135.

Yamaguchi, E., Y. Yasoshima, and T. Shimura. 2017. Systemic administration of anorexic gut peptide hormones impairs hedonic-driven sucrose consumption in mice. *Physiology & Behavior* 171:158–164.

Yun, S. P., T. I. Kam, N. Panicker, S. Kim, Y. Oh, J. S. Park, S. H. Kwon, Y. J. Park, S. S. Karuppagounder, H. Park, S. Kim, N. Oh, N. A. Kim, S. Lee, S. Brahmachari, X. Mao, J. H. Lee, M. Kumar, D. An, S. U. Kang, Y. Lee, K. C. Lee, D. H. Na, D. Kim, S. H. Lee, V. V. Roschke, S. A. Liddelow, Z. Mari, B. A. Barres, V. L. Dawson, S. Lee, T. M. Dawson, and H. S. Ko. 2018. Block of A1 astrocyte conversion by microglia is neuroprotective in models of Parkinson's disease. *Nature Medicine* 24(7):931–938.

Zang, C., H. Zhang, J. Xu, H. Zhang, S. Fouladvand, S. Havaldar, F. Cheng, K. Chen, Y. Chen, B. S. Glicksberg, J. Chen, J. Bian, and F. Wang. 2023. High-throughput target trial emulation for Alzheimer's disease drug repurposing with real-world data. *Nature Communications* 14(1):8180.

Zhang, J., T. Yi, S. Cheng, and S. Zhang. 2020. Glucagon-like peptide-1 receptor agonist exendin-4 improves neurological outcomes by attenuating TBI-induced inflammatory responses and MAPK activation in rats. *International Immunopharmacology* 86:106715.

Appendix B

Workshop Agenda

EXAMINING GLUCAGON-LIKE PEPTIDE-1 RECEPTOR (GLP-1R) AGONISTS FOR CENTRAL NERVOUS SYSTEM DISORDERS

The Keck Center, 500 Fifth Street NW
Washington, DC 20001

TUESDAY, SEPTEMBER 10, 2024
ROOM 100

9:00–9:05	Introductory Remarks **Frances Jensen**, *University of Pennsylvania*, Co-chair, Forum on Neuroscience and Nervous System Disorders **Deanna Barch**, *University of Washington in St. Louis*, Co-chair, Forum on Neuroscience and Nervous System Disorders
9:05–9:10	Workshop Overview **Matthew Hayes**, *University of Pennsylvania*, Workshop Co-chair **Brian Fiske**, *Michael J. Fox Foundation for Parkinson's Research*, Workshop Co-chair
9:10–9:25	Keynote Presentation: History of GLP-1Rs and Current Therapeutic Applications **Daniel Drucker**, *University of Toronto* (Zoom)

9:25–9:45　　Overview of GLP-1 Circuitry in the Central Nervous System
Linda Rinaman, *Florida State University*, Planning Committee Member
Anna Secher, *Novo Nordisk* (Zoom)

9:45–10:05　　Moderated Panel and Audience Q&A

SESSION 1—CLINICAL EFFICACY AND MECHANISMS OF ACTION OF GLP-1R AGONISTS IN CENTRAL NERVOUS SYSTEMS

- Review the current state of knowledge regarding the mechanisms of action of GLP-1R agonists and their therapeutic applications across different disease areas.
- Discuss available scientific evidence on the clinical efficacy of GLP-1R agonists, among other considerations, for treating various central nervous system disorders, including eating disorders, neurodegenerative diseases, and alcohol and substance use disorders.
- Consider the unique challenges (e.g., stigma, health disparities, clinical trial design, biomarker development) for each disease area.

Session 1a: Ingestive Behavior Disorders

10:05–10:10　　Session Overview
Kimberlei Richardson, *Howard University*, Session Moderator, Planning Committee Member

10:10–10:20　　A Lived Experience Utilizing GLP-1R Agonists
Patricia Nece, Obesity Action Coalition

10:20–10:45　　Speaker Presentations
Jon Davis, *Novo Nordisk*, Planning Committee Member
Elizabeth Mietlicki-Baase, *University of Buffalo*
Susan McElroy, *University of Cincinnati* (Zoom)

10:45–11:10　　Moderated Panel and Audience Q&A

11:10–11:25　　BREAK